Prozac as a Way of Life

STUDIES IN SOCIAL MEDICINE

Allan M. Brandt and Larry R. Churchill, editors

Prozac AS A WAY OF LIFE

Edited by CARL ELLIOTT and TOD CHAMBERS

THE UNIVERSITY OF NORTH CAROLINA PRESS   Chapel Hill & London

© 2004
The University of North Carolina Press
All rights reserved
Set in Cycles and Meta types
by Tseng Information Systems, Inc.
Manufactured in the United States of America

The paper in this book meets the guidelines
for permanence and durability of the Committee on
Production Guidelines for Book Longevity of the Council
on Library Resources.

Library of Congress Cataloging-in-Publication Data
Prozac as a way of life / edited by Carl Elliott and Tod
Chambers.
p. ; cm. — (Studies in social medicine)
Includes bibliographical references and index.
ISBN 0-8078-2880-7 (cloth : alk. paper) —
ISBN 0-8078-5551-0 (pbk. : alk. paper)
1. Fluoxetine—Social aspects. 2. Personality change.
[DNLM: 1. Fluoxetine—therapeutic use. 2. Bioethical Issues.
3. Depression—drug therapy. 4. Personality—drug effects.
5. Serotonin Uptake Inhibitors—therapeutic use. QV 126 P969
2004] I. Elliott, Carl, 1961- II. Chambers, Tod. III. Series.
RC483.5.F55P767 2004
616.85'27061—dc22   2003028250

cloth   08 07 06 05 04   5 4 3 2 1
paper   08 07 06 05 04   5 4 3 2 1

CONTENTS

SECTION 3
PROZAC AND THE EAST

Prozac as a Way of Life

CARL ELLIOTT

Introduction
Prozac as a Way of Life

When Peter Kramer coined the term "cosmetic psychopharmacology" in his 1993 book *Listening to Prozac*, he was referring to the way psychoactive drugs could be used not just to treat illnesses but to improve a person's psychic well-being. He described this as moving a person from one normal state to another. Like many other psychiatrists in the late 1980s and early 1990s, Kramer worried that Prozac was being used as a kind of psychic enhancement, or what other psychiatrists had called "mood brighteners." Is there anything wrong with using a drug to become "better than well"?

The term "cosmetic psychopharmacology" may have become popular with Prozac, but the concept had begun to take root in psychiatry almost forty years earlier. In 1955 Wallace Laboratories began marketing meprobamate under the trade name Miltown. Miltown has a fair claim to be the first psychoactive drug developed for the anxiety of ordinary life—or as the scientist behind the drug, Frank Berger, put it, for "people who get nervous and irritable for no good reason."[1] Unlike Thorazine (chlorpromazine), the new psychoactive drug introduced that same year for patients who were severely psychotic, Miltown was a prescription drug for the worried well. It was a biological treatment for people to whom psychiatrists would have otherwise offered psychotherapy, or maybe even no treatment at all. Miltown was marketed not as a new "sedative," like the barbiturates, but as a "tranquilizer."[2] Anxious Americans did not want to be sedated, but who could argue with a little more tranquility?

Miltown was an immediate success. Within months, demand for Miltown exceeded that of any drug ever introduced in the United States.[3] Like Prozac in the 1990s, Miltown also became a pop culture phenomenon. It was joked about on talk shows (Milton Berle called himself "Miltown Berle") and worried over in the press. The *Nation* named it a "mental laxative." *Newsweek* called it "emotional aspirin," while *Time* ran the headline, "Happiness by Prescription."[4] Psychiatrists debated whether anxiety was normal and healthy—a spur to accomplishment or creativity—or a damaging form of psychopathology for which Miltown was a legitimate treatment.

Frank Berger, the Czech physician who developed Miltown and took it to Wallace Laboratories in the early 1950s, had no such doubts himself. "Anxiety has no relation to intelligence and scholastic achievement or to the desire to achieve," Berger wrote in a celebratory 1964 issue of the *Journal of Neuropsychiatry*. Anxiety is "not a motivating force," he claimed, "but rather a symptom of disease."[5] Berger then went on to defend tranquilizers against charges that sound remarkably like those that would be leveled against Prozac thirty years later. He denied that the tranquilizers are habit forming. He denied that they are sedatives. He denied that they affect the personality, and he denied that they interfere with creativity or intellectual genius. He claimed that tranquilizers facilitate psychoanalysis and make therapy more efficient. He even downplayed any resemblance between tranquilizers and alcohol, saying, "A Miltown is no substitute for a martini."[6]

By the time Berger wrote these words in 1964, Miltown was no longer the only tranquilizer on the market. Antidepressants were available, too, but as a cultural phenomenon the antidepressants could not compare with benzodiazepines such as Librium and Valium, commonly known as "minor tranquilizers." Librium was the best-selling prescription drug of the 1960s. At the end of the decade, Valium replaced Librium in the number one spot.[7] Yet even as Frank Berger was evangelizing for tranquilizers to "liberate our minds from their primitive and outdated ways," the Rolling Stones were singing about suburban housewives who could not tolerate the mind-numbing tedium of kitchen and kids without resorting to "mother's little helpers." In the same issue of the *Journal of Neuropsychiatry* in which Berger defended the tranquilizers, writer Marya Mannes pointed out that if so many anxious Americans felt compelled to medicate themselves just so they could stand their lives, we probably ought to be asking what about their lives was producing such anxiety. For Mannes, the answer was obvious: the desire for material acquisitions and the quest for female beauty. "So great is the compulsion to acquire these things," she wrote, "so deep is the fear of their loss or lack, that the legitimate anxiety—*am I being true to myself as a human being?*—is submerged in trivia and self-deception."[8]

It is this very question—"Am I being true to myself as a human being?"—that Kramer revived in *Listening to Prozac*. Prozac, of course, was marketed as an antidepressant, not an antianxiety drug, but Kramer was struck by the way Prozac seemed to help patients whom he would not have previously thought to be clinically depressed— people who were shy, unhappy, emotionally rigid, or socially isolated. Some of these patients improved dramatically when Kramer prescribed Prozac. Yet Prozac did not sedate or tranquilize these people. Just the opposite: often it seemed to energize them. Nor did these patients merely return to their normal, baseline state. They claimed to feel better than they had ever felt before. This phenomenon Kramer called "cosmetic psychopharmacology," and he wondered whether it was the proper business of psychiatry.

Kramer noticed especially the striking language his patients were using to describe the changes they felt on Prozac. Some of them did not report feeling like a "different person" on Prozac. Instead they said they felt like themselves. "This is who I am," one patient told Kramer. "I just feel strong. I feel resilient. I feel confident."[9] Others agreed. After she went off Prozac, one woman said to him, "I am not myself."[10] She only felt like herself, she said, while taking Prozac. Remarks like these turned the old concern about cosmetic psychopharmacology on its head. It is one thing to worry that women are using psychoactive drugs to change their personalities, to tolerate their submissive social roles, or to blunt the anxiety of self-betrayal or self-deception. It is quite another matter when these same women, experiencing similar cultural pressures, say that they can become their true selves only on medication. As Kramer asked, "What are we to make of patients who navigate that culture more effectively—and achieve self-realization— on medication?"[11]

In *Listening to Prozac* Kramer was accused of exaggerating the "better than well" phenomenon, but he was far from the only psychiatrist to notice it. Arvid Carlsson of Gothenburg University in Sweden, whose work was important for the development of zimelidine, a precursor of Prozac, said, "There are people who feel so much better, who didn't have any diagnosis really. . . . I remember from the zimelidine period, that there were people whose income went up when they started to take the drug."[12] Harvard's Jonathan Cole, formerly the director of the Psychopharmacology Research Center at the National Institutes for Mental Health, says, "At McLean I treated 100 or so patients before it came on the market and a handful of them really were astoundingly better. They had been sick for 10/15 years and were clearly better than they had ever been before in their lives."[13] Roland Kuhn, the Swiss psychiatrist who first identified the antidepressant effects of imipramine to Ciba-Geigy in early 1956, claims that Prozac is now "mainly used by people who are not depressed but who use it as a pure stimulant."[14]

Clinical trials have provided evidence that the selective serotonin reuptake inhibitors (SSRIs), like other antidepressants, can effectively treat clinical depression, a potentially life-threatening condition.[15] (That evidence has also been questioned recently, with some published studies suggesting that the SSRIs are little better than placebo for depression.)[16] Yet in the decade since *Listening to Prozac* was published, the term "antidepressant" has come to seem like a very limited way to describe the SSRIs. Soon after Prozac (fluoxetine) was introduced to the American market, it was joined by Paxil (paroxetine), Luvox (fluvoxetine), Zoloft (sertraline), Effexor (venlefaxine), and Celexa (citalopram), all drugs similar in structure to Prozac. Today clinicians use the SSRIs not just for depression but also for social phobia, panic disorder, obsessive-compulsive disorder, body dysmorphic disorder, eating disorders, posttraumatic stress disorder, the impulse control disorders, Tourette's syndrome, and sexual compulsions, among many other disorders. From sex to food to body image and self-presentation, it is a rare part of ordinary American life that has not been subjected to a clinical trial involving an SSRI. GlaxoSmithKline even markets Paxil for "generalized anxiety disorder," a medical indication that takes the drugs back full circle to the days of Miltown.

One of the most striking aspects of the Prozac phenomenon is how the drug has moved out of the doctor's office and into the culture as a whole. Prozac may have begun as a brand name for fluoxetine, but it has become as recognizable and ubiquitous a brand name as Kleenex or Pampers. And like Kleenex or Pampers, Prozac has come to stand not just for a particular market item but for a type of technology: in this case, antidepressant drugs. Today when people say "Prozac," they may well be talking about any number of drugs whose brand names have never caught on in quite the same way.

Whatever the merits of the SSRIs, they have been among the most heavily promoted drugs of the past decade. The manufacturers of antidepressants have taken full advantage of the relaxation of U.S. Food and Drug Administration (FDA) restrictions on prescription drug advertising in 1997. In 2000 Paxil was the fourth most heavily promoted prescription drug in America, with $91.8 million in direct-to-consumer spending. Eli Lilly spent $37.7 million that same year advertising fluoxetine—$23.3 million as Prozac and $14.4 million as Sarafem.

To put these figures in context: GlaxoSmithKline spent more money advertising Paxil than Nike spent advertising its top shoes.[17] Direct-to-consumer advertising clearly works. From 1999 to 2000, antidepressants saw a 20.9 percent increase in sales to a figure of $10.4 billion, maintaining their position as the best-selling category of drugs in the United States. In 2000 Prozac was America's fourth most prescribed drug; Zoloft was number seven, and Paxil was number eight.[18]

Of course, the SSRIs could not have achieved such spectacular success if they did not work for some patients. Yet an equally important reason behind the success of psychoactive drugs in general, and the SSRIs in particular, is the elasticity of psychiatric diagnosis. Categories of "mental disorder" are in constant flux, and they often expand dramatically once a new treatment is marketed.[19] For example, social anxiety disorder—the fear of being embarrassed or humiliated in public—was considered a rare disorder until physicians began treating it with Nardil (phenelzine) in the mid-1980s and then, later, with SSRIs such as Paxil.[20] Today social phobia is often described as the third most common mental disorder in the United States.[21] Similar stories can be told for obsessive-compulsive disorder and panic disorder (the latter known among clinicians in the mid-1980s as the "Upjohn illness," after the makers of Xanax).[22] As David Healy has pointed out, the key to selling psychoactive drugs is to sell mental disorders.[23]

But to sell a mental disorder, you must first capture it and make it your own. A drug manufacturer is not allowed to promote a product for a specific disorder until that product has FDA approval. As a result, SSRI manufacturers jockey aggressively among themselves to claim new pieces of the mental disorder market. While the FDA has approved all six SSRIs on the market for depression, Paxil was until recently the only drug approved for social anxiety disorder. (In 2003 it was joined by Zoloft and Effexor.) All of the SSRIs except Celexa and Effexor have been approved for obsessive-compulsive disorder, but only Effexor and Paxil have been approved for generalized anxiety disorder. Zoloft and Paxil have claimed panic disorder and posttraumatic stress disorder, but only Prozac has been approved for bulimia. Eli Lilly's patent on Prozac expired in 2001, but Lilly has begun marketing the same drug under a different name, Sarafem, as a treatment for "premenstrual dysphoric disorder."

Conventional wisdom attributes the spectacular success of the SSRIs to their relative absence of side effects. For instance, monoamine oxidase inhibitors, an alternative type of antidepressant, can be dangerous without strict dietary restrictions, and people taking the longer-established tricyclic antidepressants often complain of drowsiness, dizziness, dry mouth, or constipation. Prozac and the other ssris initially appeared much less burdensome. Another significant reason for the success of the ssris lies in their ease of use. "One pill a day forever," says Jonathan Cole. "Fluoxetine at one pill a day is the ideal primary care physician's drug."[24] Today, in fact, it is no longer even one pill a day. Prozac Weekly is a once-a-week version of Prozac that Lilly has marketed using coupons in newspapers and magazines.[25] The one-pill strategy has clearly worked, whether the one pill is taken daily or weekly. It has been estimated that as much as 70 percent of the ssris is prescribed not by psychiatrists but by primary care physicians.[26]

This collection of essays has its roots in a project titled "Enhancement Technologies and Human Identity," funded by the Social Sciences and Humanities Research Council of Canada. The goal of that project was to look at medical technologies aimed not at curing illness but at improving human abilities and characteristics: "enhancement technologies," as they have come to be known. From 1997 to 2001 our multidisciplinary group met two or three times a year, often at McGill University, where the grant was based, to discuss enhancement technologies, often with several invited guests.[27] Like the essays collected here, our conversations did not concern the practical aspects of these technologies so much as the larger conceptual questions they raised.

In bioethics the conventional response to the phenomenon that Kramer called cosmetic psychopharmacology has been to classify it as an enhancement technology. The distinction between enhancement and treatment had gained currency during the ethical debate over gene therapy in the late 1980s and early 1990s. Many people were eager to press a research agenda into the therapeutic uses of genetic technology for conditions such as adenosine deaminase deficiency or cystic fibrosis but worried about the use of such technologies for eugenic purposes. Since then, bioethicists have used the term "enhancement technology" as shorthand for all sorts of technologies whose uses go beyond the strictly medical, from synthetic growth hormone for short boys to Botox injections for aging women. The unstated assumption behind the term has been that there is a morally important distinction between enhancement and treatment. Treating illness, it has been argued, is an essential part of medical practice. Doctors have an obligation to treat sick people. Enhancements, in contrast, are seen as extras—ethically acceptable, perhaps, but not something that a doctor has any particular obligation to provide or that a liberal society has an obligation to fund.

Yet the distinction between treatment and enhancement turns out to be much more elusive than it first appears, especially in psychiatry. Where is the line between psychopathology and social deviance, perversion, or eccentricity? When does shyness turn into social phobia, or melancholy into depression? The problem is complicated still further by the fact that so little is known about the causes or pathophysiology of mental disorders, or even about how chemical treatments for these mental disorders work. Philosophers have traditionally argued that illness is a departure from species-typical human functioning, but that definition offers us little guidance when the subject turns to the human mind and human behavior. What kind of behavior is typical of *Homo sapiens*?

It might be better to ask, What should we make of the social place that the SSRIs have come to occupy? Every culture has its own socially prescribed psychoactive substances, from peyote, kava, and betel nuts to alcohol, caffeine, and nicotine. But with the SSRIs, the gate to the drug is guarded by doctors, and the passport for access is the diagnosis of a mental disorder. Unlike alcohol, which is dispensed in bars and liquor stores, or caffeine, which is dispensed at Starbucks and Unitarian churches, SSRIs are dispensed at doctor's offices and pharmacies. It is the social place occupied by the SSRIs that has produced the ambivalence that many of us feel about their popularity. Unlike bartenders and espresso baristas, doctors have not generally thought of their job as making well people feel better than well. But that might change.

For the most part, our research group stayed away from questions about the distinction between enhancement and treatment. Our main interests were in identity and self-transformation. Is there anything worrying about using medication as a means of self-transformation? Is there such a thing as a true self? What does the extraordinary rise of antidepressant use over the past decade tell us about our society as a whole? The authors of the essays collected in this volume offer no unified answer to those questions; often, in fact, they disagree with one another in fundamental ways. But each essay, in its own way, addresses a question about identity. What can Prozac and its extraordinary popularity tell us about who we are and how we live now?

The essays have been divided into three sections. The first section consists of responses to some of Peter Kramer's initial questions about cosmetic psychopharmacology in *Listening to Prozac*. Some contributors to that section, such David DeGrazia and Kramer himself, are worried about what they see as misguided objections to the SSRIs, while others, such as Erik Parens and James Edwards, are concerned about the values and ways of seeing the world that an excessive reliance on SSRIs might leave behind. David Healy is concerned about how the SSRIs have been marketed and sold. The second section, with essays by Laurie Zoloth, Lauren Slater, and me, pushes the issues to other enhancement technologies and other uses for the SSRIs. The third section, with essays by Tod Chambers, Susan Squier, and Laurence Kirmayer, begins a more explicit comparison between Western psychiatric and Eastern contemplative approaches to self-transformation.

One way to begin thinking about the cultural significance of the SSRIs is to look at how late modern life pulls us in two different, often contradictory moral directions. On one hand, we have inherited a moral tradition that has come to place considerable value on the notion of authenticity.[28] Concepts such as moral integrity or self-betrayal, sincerity or duplicity, being true to yourself or selling your birthright for a mess of pottage—none of this would make any sense without the idea that we all have individual selves, that these selves have unity and integrity over time and circumstance, and that (with some qualifications) we ought to be morally committed to maintaining that unity. Even the notion of self-fulfillment, controversial though it may be, has the concept of an authentic self at its core: self-fulfillment cannot be achieved without a true self to be fulfilled. An ethic of authenticity teaches us that in order to live a meaningful life we must live a fulfilled life, and fulfillment means discovering and ultimately pursuing the values, ideals, and talents that are unique to us as individuals.

Yet this moral vocabulary has been built against a social background that encourages us to adopt a flexible, adaptable identity.[29] Contemporary life seems designed to fracture the unified self. The market requires the modern worker to be extraordinarily adaptable, able to develop new skills very quickly, willing to work on short-term contracts, and capable of "selling himself" to new employers when a position is terminated. Work life is sharply divided from leisure life, each with its own distinct customs, languages, and rituals. The Internet allows users to cultivate online personalities that can be vastly different from their real-world identities. The mass media reinforces the significance of public self-presentation at the expense of the inner, private self. With the aid of medical technology we can alter our face, body, personality, and even our sex. All of this uncertainty makes the notion of a unified, lasting, authentic self seem quaint at best and, at worst, stifling and oppressive.

The moral debate over Prozac contains some of this same tension and ambivalence about authenticity. Here is a drug that, at least according to some accounts, can help some of us become the people we want to be. By the standards of psychiatry, it allows us to "function" better. By our own moral standards, it gives us a better shot at self-fulfillment. Yet what if success is accompanied by dramatic changes — in our personality and behavior, in the way others perceive us, and in the way we make our way in the world? When we make these changes, what do we give up? This worry is by no means unique to Prozac or even to enhancement technologies more generally. It runs through much of American history: a tension between the values of self-improvement and personal achievement, on one hand, and, on the other, the values of stability, loyalty to your roots, and remembering where you came from. It should be no surprise that the language we use to describe how we feel on Prozac reflects a similar tension. We explain that Prozac has allowed us to become who we really are, even as it makes us feel different than we have ever felt before.

Does Prozac really change the self? This question is implicit in the title of Kramer's *Listening to Prozac*. Kramer suggests that by listening carefully to people who are taking a particular drug, by paying close attention to the changes in how they understand themselves, we may well come to think about the self in a very different way. If personality can change so dramatically on a drug, suggests Kramer, it is hard to avoid concluding that personality is largely a matter of biology. But such a conclusion would be premature. Prozac does not necessarily tell us anything about biology or human nature or the real nature of mental disorders. It simply tells us that some people interpret their lives and selves differently once they begin taking this drug. In the same way that a drinker may come to understand him- or herself as an alcoholic only after joining a support group, so a shy person may come to understand him- or herself as suffering from social anxiety disorder only after he or she starts taking Paxil. The drug and the disorder provide a new vocabulary with which to describe oneself. They give an individual a new way of understanding his or her history.

As the SSRIs have become more and more widely prescribed, and thus more and more a part of the popular culture, they have also helped to create new categories into which people can place themselves and understand their lives: depression, panic disorder, obsessive-compulsive disorder, and social anxiety disorder, among others. These drugs and diagnostic categories help people take what was previously a vague and inchoate set of psychic troubles and shape them into a recognizable narrative. Before taking Prozac, I may have simply thought of myself as melancholic or alienated. I may have considered myself introverted, self-conscious, and lonely. Or I may have simply found myself bewildered by the way my life had unfolded until that point. But Prozac can give me a new narrative. After I have taken Prozac, I understand that I have been suffering from a hidden clinical depression. Thus the drug gives me a new social identity.

By giving us a new way of understanding our lives, these narratives can help us make sense of events that may have previously been baffling or incoherent. In fact, if medication can correct the disorder, the mental disorder narrative may even offer the promise of a hopeful ending. But this narrative also carries a price. When we understand our problems as symptomatic of a mental disorder, we also change our moral status. While having a disorder can relieve us of the responsibility for the illness (if I have a disorder, it is not my fault), it also places new responsibilities on us. Specifically, it implies the obligation to seek psychological help. Shyness may be part of my personality, but social anxiety disorder is a potentially remediable psychiatric illness.

The mental disorder narrative need not stand up to philosophical scrutiny. All that is necessary is for the narrative to make sense to people in psychological distress. With direct-to-consumer advertising, it is enough that I see myself in the advertisements—that I feel that tingle of recognition when I see a young mother with red eyes and tear-stained cheeks, that I feel the same sense of nauseating panic that the man in the ad feels when he has to give a business presentation, or that I identify with the middle-aged homemaker who feels anxious and worried but cannot explain why.

Maybe the best way to begin to understand the cultural phenomenon that the antidepressants have become is to think about the story that drugs tell: I am the person I am, with the problems that I have, because I have this particular mental disorder. It is a story that provides me with a sympathetic listener (my doctor or therapist), a community of like-minded sufferers (my support group), and a coherent narrative (told on television) both for myself and for those to whom I must explain myself. Increasingly, this is a story of biology and the brain, in which biological psychiatrists, pharmaceutical companies, and patient support groups all agree that disorders that respond to the SSRIS must have biological roots. Eventually this story may even cre-

Introduction

ate a new set of criteria for what counts as an acceptable identity, one of which will be response to treatment. If I am to be admitted to the community of social phobia, anxiety, or clinical depression, my identity papers must certify that I have responded to an antidepressant.

The story of how this volume came about might have stopped at this point. But in the spring of 2000 the *Hastings Center Report* published a special issue titled "Prozac, Alienation and the Self," which included abbreviated versions of the essays in this volume written by David DeGrazia, James Edwards, David Healy, Peter Kramer, and me. Four of those essays had been previously presented at meetings of the Enhancement Technologies Group, while DeGrazia had submitted his essay to the *Report* independently. Several months after the essays appeared, the Hastings Center received a letter from a representative of the Eli Lilly Corporation, the manufacturer of Prozac and the Hastings Center's largest annual corporate donor. In that letter Lilly announced that it would no longer be making its annual financial contribution to the Hastings Center.[30] Laurel Swartz, manager of corporate communications for Eli Lilly, later explained it this way: "The center had published articles that Lilly felt contained information that was biased and scientifically unfounded and that may have led to significant misinformation to readers, patients and the community."[31]

While Lilly's annual $25,000 contribution was not large by industry standards, its withdrawal provoked much self-examination at the Hastings Center and elsewhere, particularly around the role of corporate funding in bioethics scholarship. What would it mean for the field if bioethicists were forced to risk financial punishment whenever they criticized corporate policy? In the spring of 2001 the *Hastings Center Report* featured a symposium called "Bioethics in Business," devoted to corporate funding of bioethics. In it a number of commentators, including me, alternately criticized and defended the practice of bioethicists accepting funding from the pharmaceutical industry.[32]

The controversy did not end there. In November 2000 David Healy gave a presentation on the history of psychopharmacology at the Centre for Addiction and Mental Health (CAMH), an affiliate hospital of the University of Toronto. Healy is a psychopharmacologist, a practicing psychiatrist, and a historian of psychiatry at the University of Wales. It was Healy's paper in the *Hastings Center Report*, "Good Science or Good Business?" that had attracted the brunt of Eli Lilly's criticism—in particular his brief remarks about a possible association between antidepressants and suicide. In his Toronto talk, as in his paper in the *Hastings Center Report*, Healy briefly mentioned his worries that in rare cases, Prozac could result in a higher risk of suicide or violence.[33]

Shortly thereafter, the CAMH rescinded Healy's appointment. He was not told why the appointment was being withdrawn or why the CAMH suddenly changed its mind about a job for which it had assiduously courted him for more than a year. Healy was simply informed by e-mail that the CAMH did not feel that his "approach was compatible with the goals for development of the academic and clinical resource" of the clinic. As it happens, the CAMH is the recipient of a $1.5-million gift from Eli Lilly. The Mood Disorders Program, which Healy was to direct, receives 52 percent of its funding from corporate sources.[34]

The CAMH publicly denied that corporate funding had anything to do with its decision to rescind Healy's appointment. Yet in the absence of any other credible explanation of its sudden turnaround, that denial struck many observers as a little hollow. The Canadian Association of University Teachers issued statements in strong support of Healy, suggesting that in rescinding the offer, the CAMH had breached Healy's academic freedom. A letter protesting the actions of the CAMH was signed by an international group of twenty-seven neuropharmacologists, including past presidents of the American College of Neuropsychopharmacology, the European Association of Psychiatrists, and the American Psychiatric Association.[35] In September 2001 Healy filed a $9.4 million (Can) lawsuit against the University of Toronto and the CAMH for breach of contract and libel. In April 2002 that suit was settled out of court.[36]

Why such controversy over an academic presentation? Both the Hastings Center and CAMH episodes must be understood in light of a decade of debate about whether the SSRIs can increase the risk of suicide or violence. In 1990 the *American Journal of Psychiatry* published a paper by Harvard University's Martin Teicher and colleagues titled "Emergence of Intense Suicidal Preoccupation during Fluoxetine [Prozac] Treatment," which described a number of patients who became agitated, obsessed with violence, and suicidal shortly after starting Prozac.[37] Similar case reports and discussions appeared in other journals, including the *New England Journal of Medicine*.[38] The *Lancet* published a favorable editorial on the SSRIs that nonetheless warned that they could promote suicidal thoughts and behavior.[39] Newsmagazines and talk shows began running stories on Prozac and suicide, and costly lawsuits were filed against Eli Lilly.[40] Lilly quickly offered to pay all legal expenses for any physician sued for prescribing Prozac.[41]

Introduction

When these reports began to appear in the media, the FDA assembled a committee of independent experts to look into the question of suicide, violence, and the SSRIs. After a one-day hearing in September 1991, the committee issued a report stating that it had found no credible evidence to suggest that the SSRIs caused suicidal or violent impulses.[42] Yet the FDA report did not settle the suicide controversy, because many outside observers saw the "independent" committee appointed by the FDA as anything but independent. According to Joseph Glenmullen's book *Prozac Backlash*, five of the nine members of the committee had financial ties to the pharmaceutical industry. The FDA had waived its own conflict-of-interest policy so that these members could participate. Of six consultants appointed to advise the committee, four required waivers of the conflict-of-interest policy. Half of the formal presentations to the committee were made by representatives of Eli Lilly.[43]

Thirteen years later, opinion about antidepressants seems to be turning against the industry. In 2001 a Wyoming jury awarded $6.4 million to the family of a man who had shot his wife, daughter, and granddaughter before killing himself while taking Paxil.[44] (Healy testified as an expert witness in that trial.) Three years later, British regulators banned the use of Paxil (called Seroxat in the United Kingdom) for people under age eighteen after discovering that GlaxoSmithKline's own data (most of which had not been published or made available to regulators) showed that children taking Paxil were more than three times as likely as those taking placebo to harm themselves or have suicidal thoughts. Soon afterward the FDA recommended that doctors stop prescribing Paxil to people under eighteen. Questions have also been raised about how forthcoming Eli Lilly has been to regulators about Prozac. Court records have shown that Lilly never informed the FDA that German regulators initially refused to approve the sale of Prozac in 1985 because of concerns over a link with suicide. According to the *New York Times*, many of the members of the FDA panel that cleared Prozac in 1991 now say they would reconsider that decision.[45]

The irony of our research group getting mixed up with the suicide controversy, of course, is that our interest was not in Prozac's side effects but in its success. We were interested in the *good* results. Yet the financial stakes involved in the Prozac controversy are so high and so pervasive that brushups with industry have become increasingly difficult to avoid. Many academic psychiatrists and university departments of psychiatry depend for their livelihood on funding from the pharmaceutical and biotechnology industries. Today psychiatrists

conduct clinical trials for industry, enter patent and royalty agree-
ments with industry, serve as industry consultants and members of
industry advisory boards, accept gifts from industry, travel to exotic
locations at industry expense, accept generous honoraria for industry-
sponsored lectures, sign their names to ghostwritten articles for industry, and even hold industry stock.[46] Marcia Angell, the former editor of the *New England Journal of Medicine*, has written that when the
journal published an article in 2000 on the antidepressants, the ties
of its authors to the drug industry were so extensive that the journal
did not have sufficient space to list them all in print and was forced
to run them on its Web site instead. When Angell decided to commis-
sion an editorial on the issue, she could find very few who did not have
financial ties to the makers of antidepressants.[47]

In light of the controversy over Healy's "Good Science or Good
Business?" we have decided to reprint the article here just as it appeared in the *Hastings Center Report*. (Healy has published a postscript
to the article in *Perspectives in Biology and Medicine*, explaining the
background to the controversy over Prozac and suicide and the series
of events that followed its publication.) While academic book pub-
lishers have generally not required authors to disclose their financial
conflicts of interest, we decided that it would also be best if we asked
the contributors to this book to disclose any financial association with
the pharmaceutical or biotechnology industry, as well as any other financial affiliations that might compromise the quality or objectivity of
their manuscripts. Any disclosures that the authors made are included
at the end of each essay.

NOTES

1. Quoted in Edward Shorter, *A History of Psychiatry: From the Era of the
Asylum to the Age of Prozac* (New York: John Wiley and Sons, 1997), 315.

2. See the interview with Paul Janssen, founder of Janssen Pharmaceuticals, in *The Psychopharmacologists II: Interviews by David Healy*, ed. David
Healy (London: Altman, 1998), 59.

3. Shorter, *History of Psychiatry*, 316.

4. Mickey Smith, *Small Comfort: A History of Minor Tranquilizers* (New
York: Praeger), 69–74.

5. Frank Berger, "The Tranquilizer Decade," *Journal of Neuropsychiatry* 5
(1964): 407.

6. Ibid., 406.

7. Shorter, *History of Psychiatry*, 319.

8. Marya Mannes, "The Roots of Anxiety in the Modern Woman," *Journal of Neuropsychiatry* 5 (1964): 412.

9. Peter D. Kramer, *Listening to Prozac* (London: Fourth Estate, 1994), 219.

10. Ibid., 19.

11. Ibid., 294.

12. Healy, *Psychopharmacologists II*, 77.

13. Ibid., 259.

14. Ibid., 114.

15. For reviews of the literature, see Olav Spigest and Bjorn Martensson, "Fortnightly Review: Drug Treatment of Depression," *British Medical Journal* 318 (May 1, 1999): 1188–91; John R. Geddes, Nick Freemantle, James Mason, Martin P. Eccles, and Janette Boynton, "Selective Serotonin Reuptake Inhibitors for Depression," Cochrane Database of Systematic Reviews, Cochrane Library, updated August 29, 2001.

16. Irving Kirsch, Thomas J. Moore, Alan Scoboria, and Sara S. Nicholls, "The Emperor's New Drugs: An Analysis of Antidepressant Medication Data Submitted to the U.S. Food and Drug Administration," *Prevention and Treatment* 5, article 23, posted July 15, 2002; Hypericum Depression Trial Study Group, "Effect of Hypericum Perforatum (St. John's Wort) in Major Depressive Disorder: A Randomized Controlled Trial," *Journal of the American Medical Association* 287 (2002): 1807–14.

17. National Institute for Health Care Management, "Prescription Drugs and Mass Media Drugs Advertising" (2000), 9 (available at <www.nihcm.org>).

18. These figures come from National Institute for Health Care Management, "Prescription Drug Expenditures in 2000: The Upward Trend Continues" (available at <www.nihcm.org>); see esp. pp. 17 and 19.

19. Allan V. Horwitz, *Creating Mental Illness* (Chicago: University of Chicago Press, 2002).

20. M. R. Liebowitz, A. J. Fyer, J. M. Gorman, R. Campeas, and A. Levin, "Phenelzine in Social Phobia," *Journal of Clinical Psychopharmacology* 6, no. 2 (1986): 93–98; M. R. Liebowitz, J. M. Gorman, A. J. Fyer, R. Campeas, A. P. Levin, D. Sandberg, E. Hollander, L. Papp, and D. Goetz, "Pharmacotherapy of Social Phobia: An Interim Report of a Placebo-Controlled Comparison of Phenelzine and Atenolol," *Journal of Clinical Psychiatry* 49, no. 7 (1988): 252–57; M. R. Liebowitz, F. Schneier, R. Campeas, J. Gorman, A. Fyer, E. Hollander, J. Hatterer, and L. Papp, "Phenelzine and Atenolol in Social Phobia," *Psychopharmacology Bulletin* 26, no. 1 (1990): 123–25; M. B. Stein, M. R. Liebowitz, R. B. Lydiard, C. D. Pitts, W. Bushnell, and I. Gergel, "Paroxetine Treatment of Generalized Social Phobia (Social Anxiety Disorder): A Ran-

domized Controlled Trial," *Journal of the American Medical Association* 280, no. 8 (1998): 708–13; D. Baldwin, J. Bobes, D. J. Stein, I. Scharwachter, and M. Faure, "Paroxetine in Social Phobia/Social Anxiety Disorder: Random-ised, Double-Blind, Placebo-Controlled Study," Paroxetine Study Group, *British Journal of Psychiatry* 175 (1999): 120–26.

21. Ronald C. Kessler, Katherine A. McGonagle, et al., "Lifetime and 12-Month Prevalence of DSM-III-R Psychiatric Disorders in the United States: Results from the National Comorbidity Survey," *Archives of General Psychia-try* 51, no. 1 (1994): 8–19; Lynne Lamberg, "Social Phobia: Not Just Another Name for Shyness," *Journal of the American Medical Association* 280, no. 8 (August 26, 1998): 685–86.

22. Shorter, *History of Psychiatry*, 320.

23. David Healy, *The Antidepressant Era* (Cambridge, Mass.: Harvard University Press, 1997).

24. Healy, *Psychopharmacologists II*, 259.

25. Vanessa O'Connell and Rachel Zimmerman, "Drug Pitches Resonate with Edgy Public," *Wall Street Journal*, January 14, 2002.

26. M. J. Grinfeld, "Protecting Prozac," *California Lawyer*, December 1998, 36–40, 79; E. J. Pollock, "Managed Care's Focus on Psychiatric Drugs Alarms Many Doctors," *Wall Street Journal*, December 1, 1995. These citations come from Joseph Glenmullen, *Prozac Backlash* (New York: Touchstone, 2000), 17.

27. Members of the project were Francoise Baylis (philosophy, Dalhousie University); Tod Chambers (religious studies, Northwestern University); Alice Dreger (history and philosophy of science, Michigan State Univer-sity); Carl Elliott (philosophy and medicine, University of Minnesota); David Gems (genetics, University College London); Kathy Glass (law, Mc-Gill University); Lawrence Kirmayer (psychiatry, McGill University); and Margaret Lock (anthropology, McGill University).

28. The classic text here is Lionel Trilling, *Sincerity and Authenticity* (Cam-bridge, Mass.: Harvard University Press, 1982). See also Charles Taylor's *Sources of the Self* (Cambridge, Mass.: Harvard University Press, 1989).

29. Kenneth Gergen, *The Saturated Self* (New York: Basic Books, 1990); Robert Jay Lifton, *The Protean Self* (Chicago: University of Chicago Press, 1999).

30. Greg Kaebnick, "What About the Report?," *Hastings Center Report* 31, no. 2 (March–April 2001): 16–17.

31. Anne McIlroy, "Prozac Critic Sees U of T Job Revoked," *Toronto Globe and Mail*, April 14, 2001.

32. *Hastings Center Report* 31, no. 2 (March–April 2001): 9–21.

33. That talk was been posted on the Web site of the journal *Nature Medi-cine* and can still be seen at <http://wwtiv.pharmapolitics.com/>.

34. This statistic was reported on the Canadian Broadcasting Service news documentary program *The National* on July 11, 2001. The documentary can be seen online on the service's Web site at <http://cbc.ca/national/real/ nightly_national.smil>. A detailed chronicle of the CAMH affair was also published in Sarah Boseley, "Bitter Pill," *Guardian* (United Kingdom), May 7, 2001.

35. See Karen Birchard "Scientists Worldwide Protest Withdrawal of Job Offer at U. of Toronto," *Chronicle of Higher Education*, September 11, 2001; Owen Dyer, "University Accused of Violating Academic Freedom to Safe-guard Funding from Drug Companies," *British Medical Journal* 323 (September 15, 2001): 591.

36. Constance Holden, "Drug Critic Sues after School Pulls Job Offer," *Science*, October 5, 2001, 29–30; Julie Smyth, "Psychiatrist Denied Job Sues U of T: Linked Prozac to Suicide," *National Post* (Canada), September 25, 2001.

37. M. H. Teicher, C. Glod, and J. O. Cole, "Emergence of Intense Suicidal Preoccupation during Fluoxetine Treatment," *American Journal of Psychiatry* 147 (1990): 207–10.

38. P. Masand, S. Gupta, and N. I. Dewan, "Suicidal Ideation Related to Fluoxetine Treatment," *New England Journal of Medicine* 324 (February 7, 1991): 420. See also H. Koizumi, "Fluoxetine and Suicidal Ideation," *Journal of the American Academy of Child and Adolescent Psychiatry* 30 (1991): 695; J. J. Mann and S. Kapur, "The Emergence of Suicidal Ideation and Behavior during Antidepressant Pharmacotherapy," *Archives of General Psychiatry* 48, no. 11 (1991): 1027–33; R. A. King, M. A. Riddle, P. B. Chappell, et al., "Emergence of Self-Destructive Phenomena in Children and Adolescents during Fluoxetine Treatment," *Journal of the American Academy of Child and Adolescent Psychiatry* 30 (1991): 179–86; K. Dasgupta, "Additional Cases of Suicidal Ideation Associated with Fluoxetine," *American Journal of Psychiatry* 147 (1990): 1570; L. A. Papp and J. M. Gorman, "Suicidal Preoccupation during Fluoxetine Treatment," *American Journal of Psychiatry* 147 (1990): 1380.

39. Editorial, "5-HT Blockers and All That," *Lancet*, August 11, 1990, 345.

40. N. Angier, "Eli Lilly Facing Million-Dollar Suits on Its Antidepressant Drug Prozac," *New York Times*, August 16, 1990.

41. A. D. Marcus and W. Lambert, "Eli Lilly to Pay Costs of Doctors after They Prescribe Prozac," *Wall Street Journal*, June 6, 1991; M. Mitka, "Drug Maker to Defend Physicians Sued over Prozac," *American Medical News*, June 14, 1991.

42. T. Burton, "Panel Finds No Credible Evidence to Tie Prozac to Suicides and Violent Behavior," *Wall Street Journal*, September 23, 1991.

43. Glenmullen, *Prozac Backlash*, 156–58.

44. Philip J. Hilts, "Jury Awards $6.4 Million in Killings Tied to Drug," *New York Times*, June 8, 2001.

45. Sarah Boseley, "Mood Drug Seroxat Banned for Under-18s," *Guardian*, June 11, 2003; Katherine Lutz, *Boston Globe*, August 5, 2003; Gardiner Harris, "Debate Resumes on the Safety of Depression's Wonder Drugs," *New York Times*, August 7, 2003.

46. Marcia Angell and Arnold S. Relman, "Prescription for Profit," *Washington Post*, June 20, 2001; Sarah Boseley, "Scandal of Scientists Who Take Money for Papers Ghostwritten by Drug Companies: Doctors Named as Authors May Not Have Seen Raw Data," *Guardian*, February 7, 2002; Sheryl Stolberg, "Scientists Often Mum about Ties to Industry," *New York Times*, April 25, 2001; Julie Appleby, "Sales Pitch: Drug Firms Use Perks to Push Pills," *USA Today*, May 16, 2001; Richard Horton, "Lotronex and the FDA: A Fatal Erosion of Integrity," *Lancet*, May 19, 2001, 1544–45; Sarah Boseley, "Psychiatric Agenda 'Set By Drug Firms,'" *Guardian Unlimited*, July 9, 2001. In 2000 the *Journal of the American Medical Association* devoted a thematic issue to conflict of interest. See *Journal of the American Medical Association* 284, no. 17 (2000): 2143–2276.

47. Marcia Angell, "Is Academic Medicine for Sale?," *New England Journal of Medicine* 342 (May 18, 2000): 1516–18. See also Boseley, "Scandal of Scientists Who Take Money for Papers."

SECTION 1
Responses to Prozac from Philosophy and Psychiatry

Kramer's Anxiety

In the very first paragraph of *Listening to Prozac*, Peter Kramer presents the case of Sam, a melancholic and proudly unconventional architect.[1] Kramer explains that a central conflict in Sam's marriage was his interest in pornographic videos. Despite his wife's distaste, Sam insisted that she watch hard-core sex films with him.

We learn that after a reversal in his business and the death of his parents, Sam became depressed. He came to understand his depression in terms of those unhappy events, but that did not make him feel better. Eventually Kramer prescribed Prozac, and Sam underwent a remarkable transformation. Suddenly he could complete projects in one draft; he could remember more and concentrate better. He was more poised. He could speak at professional meetings without notes.

Though Sam now reported feeling "better than well," one part of his transformation troubled him. He no longer was interested in pornography, and that change felt like a loss. According to Kramer, "The style he had nurtured and defended for years now seemed not part of him but an illness." A part of his self that once seemed essential now seemed alien. Kramer continues: "Although he was grateful for the relief Prozac gave him from his mental anguish, this one aspect of his recovery was disconcerting, *because the medication redefined what was essential and what contingent about his own personality—and the drug agreed with his wife when she was being critical*" (11, my emphasis).

The part of that sentence before the dash telegraphs the book's central questions: What are we doing when we "listen to drugs," when we allow them to tell us which "parts" of our self are essential and which are not? What are we doing when we allow drugs to teach us that this aspect of our self is authentic and that one alien? Which conceptions of authenticity inform those discriminations? That is, are we allowing drugs to teach us oppressive—or liberatory—conceptions of what it is to be and become an authentic self? Most specifically, are we allowing drugs like Prozac to teach us oppressive or liberatory views of what it is for women to be and become "authentic"?

Those questions about authenticity in general and of women in particular are the source of what I will call Kramer's anxiety. Kramer is, after all, a physician, who has to decide what drugs to prescribe, to whom, and when. As a thinker, he is keenly aware of medicine's history of pathologizing behaviors that subsequently came to be seen as healthy but different (e.g., homosexuality) or as healthy responses to unjust situations (e.g., anomie in the face of domestic purgatory). As a physician and a thinker, Kramer is anxious about the possibility that in prescribing Prozac, he is sometimes being complicit with unjust or arbitrary conceptions of persons in general and women in particular. (Please note: Kramer is not anxious about using Prozac to treat clinical depression, nor am I.)

The part of that sentence after the dash ("and the drug agreed with [Sam's] wife when she was being critical") foreshadows Kramer's response to those questions regarding Prozac and authenticity. It foreshadows the line of argument he hopes will cure his anxiety. That argument suggests that Prozac does not necessarily promote oppressive views of the self. More specifically, if anything, Prozac promotes liberatory views, even what Kramer calls "feminist" views. Prozac agrees with Sam's wife—and presumably "feminists": watching pornography is not only hurtful to women, it is not an essential part of a healthy man; it is something alien, something inauthentic. So if we are listening to Prozac, we need not be anxious. If anything, according to Kramer's anxiolytic argument, Prozac promotes a "feminist" conception of the authentic self.

My point here is not to suggest that Kramer and Prozac are wrong about pornography. I am not saying that Prozac hurt Sam in depriving him of his authentic desire to watch pornography. I am as New Age and sensitive a guy as you are likely to meet. My point is not about pornography at all. It is that from the very beginning of his book, Kramer goes to great pains to suggest that we—and he—need not be anxious about what Prozac will teach us regarding the authenticity of persons in general and women in particular.

Kramer does indeed speak throughout the book about Prozac in terms like the ones he uses to describe Sam: Prozac can help to *discover* the *authentic* self, which lies just beneath the surface of environmental assault and genetic bad luck. Like many of us, however, Kramer thinks and speaks at different times in different terms about the self. In fact, when he makes his most concerted attempt to assuage his anxiety about what we are doing when we listen to Prozac, he does not rely on the notion of the self as that which we *discover*. For the sorts of good reasons suggested by David DeGrazia in his essay in this book, Kramer does not stand solely by the view that there is an authentic self to discover.[2] Ultimately, what assuages Kramer's anxiety is the view that Prozac facilitates *an authentic process* of self *creation*. Prozac, he argues, does not promote or teach any dominant view of what the authentic self is. *Prozac* does not, to borrow from the language of his subtitle, "remake the self." *We*, Kramer argues, use Prozac to remake ourselves according to our own lights.

In this essay I explore in more detail the two conceptions of the self that Kramer appeals to when he makes his case that Prozac promotes the authenticity of people in general and women in particular. I explore the assumptions he makes and the questions he downplays on the way to assuaging his anxiety. In the end, I suggest why Kramer's cure will not work.

DISCOVERING THE SELF WITH PROZAC

The first (right-hand) page of a recent three-page ad for Prozac's chemical cousin, Paxil, presents the image of a huge rock, in which the reader sees a not-yet-finished sculpture. Already visible are the torso, arms, and face of a man whose longing for liberation from the rock is palpable. From what is already visible, the reader can easily imagine how the whole man will look. On the ad's next two glossy pages we see the man fully emerged and exultant. Paxil is the chisel that allowed him to spring free and whole from his prison.

That conception of authenticity—there is a self that just needs to be discovered or freed from life's inessential encrustations—is a great hook for selling drugs. That way of thinking about the self and about what Prozac can do to uncover it (remember Sam's inauthentic fondness for porn) does not only appeal to Kramer. It also often appeals to his patients.

Tess is the first character Kramer introduces in detail. Though her life was strewn with trauma and sorrow, she managed to learn to nurture others, including her employees, siblings, and mother. She made remarkable adjustments and adaptations in the face of horrendous odds, but her unhappiness eventually brought her to Kramer's office. When Kramer first diagnosed her depression and prescribed imipramine, her response was great. Once on imipramine, Tess reported, "I am myself again" (4).

According to Kramer, while she was on imipramine, Tess no longer met the criteria for depression. But as he puts it, he was not yet satisfied, because he thought he picked up "a soft sign or two of depression," and he worried that Tess was at risk for relapse. Further, subtle concerns about Tess's difficulty in both her work and romantic worlds moved Kramer to increase the imipramine. But due to unpleasant side effects, he decided to prescribe Prozac. Kramer explains that his purpose was to "restore" Tess to her "premorbid self."

Much to his astonishment, however, she was not restored but "transformed." Whereas before she snuck around with abusive, married men, now she had three dates a weekend with the kinds of guys any gal would love to bring home to meet Mom and Dad. Whereas before she tended to evade confrontation at work, now she took the bull by the horns. Not only did her company's troubles settle down, but she got a big raise. She lost weight, her humor improved, and she even was freed up to attempt a rapprochement with her mother. After Tess's extraordinary response, in keeping with the usual protocol, Kramer tried to wean her off the medication.

Eight months after she stopped the Prozac, Tess phoned Kramer and reported, "I am not myself" (18). As the drug companies would have her, Tess speaks as if the drug helped to uncover her true self. She asks for more of the drug so she can restore that recently discovered self. Kramer, however, acknowledges—again, the whole book attempts to come to terms with the fact—that Tess learned the contours of her "authentic self" from the drug. As Kramer tells us at length, the drug's power to affect the self worried him: "I was torn simultaneously by a sense that the medication was too far-reaching . . . and a sense that my discomfort was arbitrary and aesthetic rather than doctorly. I wondered how the drug might influence my profession's definition of illness and its understanding of ordinary suffering. I wondered how Prozac's success would interact with certain unfortunate tendencies of the broader culture" (20). To assuage those worries Kramer adopts a complementary—and perhaps more compelling—conception of authenticity than the one suggested by the Paxil ad and Tess's words.

CREATING THE SELF WITH PROZAC

Instead of asking, Does a drug like Prozac help one to discover her authentic self? the complementary strategy asks, Does Prozac promote an authentic process by which one can shape her self? What the two

ERIK PARENS

strategies share is the aim of showing that Prozac is the friend of authenticity and liberation in general—and women in particular.

Kramer's second major case involves Julia, a married registered nurse with children. Julia does part-time paid work so she can be home at the end of the school day to do the unpaid work of caring for her children. She suffers from perfectionism, which was "so pronounced that she was continually angry at her children and husband and, given the impossibility of instilling her standards in them, [she was] stalemated in her career." Though Kramer initially was reluctant to prescribe a drug to someone he saw as struggling with a combination of context-dependent psychosocial issues and with symptoms that perhaps fell in the penumbra of obsessive-compulsive disorder, he prescribed Prozac.

Like Tess, Julia felt that her life was transformed when on Prozac; when off it, she reported, "I don't feel myself" (29). When off the drug, she did not feel as assertive, resilient, and confident as when on it. At this juncture in the book Kramer worries at length about whether he is using Prozac to do for Julia what doctors did in the 1960s when they prescribed Valium. In retrospect we see that those 1960s physicians prescribed Valium to help women endure patently unjust social arrangements and attitudes. Kramer wonders whether fifty years from now the same charge might be leveled against doctors such as himself.

He worries that he and other doctors are prescribing a drug to help people live up to dominant ideals that are, if not patently unjust, then surely arbitrary. He recognizes that, for example, when he was a child, his German-born female relatives prized the very sort of "perfectionism" that now makes Julia's life so difficult. He appreciates John Updike's observation that "masochism [in women] is as unfashionable now as aggressiveness was twenty years ago" (40). Later in the book, when he returns to this same worry, he recognizes that bereavement considered pathological in the United States would be considered quite healthy in a country like Greece, where normal grieving takes five years. As well as anybody, Kramer understands the concern about using Prozac to promote culturally specific, currently fashionable conceptions of the self.

One of his responses to that worry is to point out that physicians and persons who suffer do not have the luxury of speculating about whether the values they measure themselves against are just or not, arbitrary or not. They do not have the luxury of speculating about the extent to which cultural values are relative. "In the everyday practice of medicine, and in the everyday valuation of human success and suffering, it is fruitless to try to maintain the viewpoint of cultural relativism" (41). If somebody is suffering as a result of not living up to current norms, then those with the means to do so are obliged to respond. On that view, it is at best silly to worry that giving a patient a drug to better approximate current cultural norms is a problem. People who suffer want and deserve relief, not finger wagging about the need for cultural change.

The second and far more developed—and more powerful—response to that worry is that this particular drug, Prozac, could be used in any time to help any person to create her own self. This drug is different from drugs that produce particular ways of being. It can help anybody create her own life projects, whatever they may be, in whatever way she sees fit. Prozac is "the opposite of mother's little helper [i.e., Valium]: it got Julia out of the house and into the workplace." Kramer avers, "There is a sense in which antidepressants are feminist drugs, liberating and empowering" (40).

Those who worry that Prozac *makes* assertive and sunny selves of a particular "virile," American variety are, Kramer suggests, confused. They think Prozac is a "mood brightener." But it is not. Prozac does not make or mask moods; it does not keep people from seeing life the way it really is. It does not "rob life of the edifying potential for tragedy." Rather, he argues, "it catalyzes the precondition for tragedy, namely participation." Nor does Prozac promote self-absorption (like marijuana or LSD). It promotes other-directed, social activities. As Kramer puts it, Prozac "generally increases personal autonomy" (265).

At this crucial juncture in his argument, Kramer suggests that Prozac does not transform selves. Instead, Prozac frees persons so that they can transform themselves. Indeed, at the end of the book Kramer suggests that the ideal psychiatrist of the future is embodied by Dr. Yang in Woody Allen's movie *Alice*. In that movie, the sage Dr. Yang uses a combination of drugs and words to help Alice transform herself. "His drugs potentiate change; ultimately, it is Alice's quest that transforms" (290).

IS PROZAC A MORALLY NEUTRAL TECHNOLOGY?

Thus, to relieve his anxiety about whether in prescribing Prozac he inadvertently complies with patently unjust or simply arbitrary conceptions of the self, Kramer makes a familiar move. (I surely have made it.) Like any technology, goes the argument, Prozac can be put to good or bad purposes; "in itself" it is morally neutral. Though Prozac *can* be used by people who want to better approximate dominant norms, it *need not* be used for that purpose. As Kramer puts it in his essay in this volume, "If Prozac induces conformity, it is to an ideal of assertiveness, but assertiveness can be in the service of social reform of the sort ordinarily understood as nonconformity or rebellion."[3] Just like fire can be used to cook food or annihilate one's enemies, Prozac can be used to facilitate social conformity or rebellion.

In more nuanced terms than mine, Jim Edwards suggests in his essay in this volume that there is an old and important debate between those who are most impressed by the extent to which we freely choose to put technology to whatever purposes we see fit and those who are most impressed by the extent to which the very existence of a technology bounds and shapes our choices.[4] Given that both sides of that debate harbor insights about different aspects of technology, it is not surprising that sometimes we find it useful to think of technology in one way and then in the other: now as neutral and then as reality shaping.

It is surprising, however, to see Kramer rely so heavily on the technology-is-neutral view, given that one of his greatest contributions is to show how Prozac can shape—even "transform"—what we understand a self to be. It is he who teaches that because we have "listened to Prozac," where once we saw normal human variation ("melancholy") now we see pathology ("dysthymia"). The technology has taught us how to see the world differently and, in so doing, has transformed it. Prozac created a purpose where once there was none (different from melancholy, dysthymia requires intervention). On this other view of technology, drugs like Prozac are not just tools; they are part of the frame; they shape how and what we see and want.

Moreover, the technology-is-neutral view invites us to ignore that in this culture Prozac is now being used—and predictably will be used—in very particular ways. Perhaps Prozac *could* be used to promote projects of rebellion. But no one I am aware of has provided credible evidence to suggest that it *is* being used for such purposes. Certainly Kramer does not. On the contrary, he provides abundant evidence that the drug helps his patients better approximate the currently fashionable ideal of the assertive, confident, resilient, romantically satisfied producer and consumer.

Kramer's suggestion that Prozac is a morally neutral tool that we can use to shape our selves and life projects according to our own lights is problematic in another respect. When we ask along with Kramer, Does the drug liberate people to craft their selves and life projects as they see fit? we may let ourselves off the hook of asking, Liberation *for what kinds of life?* When we ask, Does the drug help us to discover and/or create ourselves? we may let ourselves off the hook of asking, *What kinds* of selves are we discovering and/or creating? What kinds of selves and life projects are we turning toward—and away from?

Though he may downplay those questions, to his credit Kramer does not ignore them. He does identify some of the personality traits—and thus sorts of selves—that Prozac turns us away from (and toward). It makes Kramer anxious to see the drug sometimes inadvertently diminish traits such as "seriousness," "subtlety," and "sensitivity."

In the first chapter, in his presentation of Tess, the woman who gives too much, Kramer explains that when she took Prozac, her relationship to those she had previously cared for changed. "She was no longer drawn to tragedy, nor did she feel heightened responsibility for the injured." Not only did her internal states change, but so did her address; she moved to a nearby town, farther from her mother than she had ever been. As Kramer observes, "Whether these last changes are to be applauded depends on one's social values. Tess's guilty vigilance over a mother about whom she had strong ambivalent feelings can be seen as a virtue, one that medication helped to erode. Tess experienced her 'loss of seriousness,' as she put it, as a relief. She had been too devoted in the past, at too great a cost to her own enjoyment in life" (9). To ignore the gender inequities that get played out in some forms of "seriousness" would be a bad mistake. To ignore the reality of masochism would be foolish.

But to ignore that we live in a culture where seriousness increasingly takes too long and earns too little is equally foolish. Many parts of our lives—the parts increasingly hidden away by our dominant ways of being—shout out for seriousness. The suffering of our neighbors calls out for seriousness. So does the destruction of our habitat. So does our mortality. Seriousness can, of course, as Nietzsche would have it, smell bad. Sometimes it is no more than resentment masquerading. Sometimes it squashes joy. But it would be a mistake to ignore that we live in a culture where seriousness itself increasingly gets squashed. It does not make anyone appear younger or prettier. It does not sell.

In another case, Kramer describes Gail, who used shopping for clothes and a variety of drugs "to treat or head off a succession of ill-defined bad feelings" (93). Prozac helped. Like Sam, Gail, too, could begin making presentations at professional meetings without notes. But when the chairmanship of a hospital department opened up, she asked Kramer if he would increase her dose so that she might have the confidence to throw her hat in the ring. Kramer acceded to her request. She did not get the job, "but she was able to take the rebuff in stride." Moreover, her marriage improved. "Though Gail's need to dress perfectly may have diminished, she held on to her right to spend money on herself as a badge and an instrument of independence, and as a bargaining chip in her marriage. If anything she enjoyed shopping more. 'I don't feel guilty about spending,' she said. 'My husband can say what he wants'" (95). To ignore that guilt can siphon off pleasure from life would be foolish. We can both understand that and ask, Will it be good for our selves and our society if more of us feel less guilty about spending and consuming? It is quicker and easier to satisfy the desire for consumption than the desire for connection with others or the desire for meaningful work.

Kramer, whose life appears to be devoted to connection with others and meaningful work, of course does not think that spending guilt-lessly will make us happier. Guiltless spending is a side effect, not the intended effect of Prozac. But it is a side effect that meshes seamlessly with what can be one of the drug's primary uses: to facilitate better performance in an often cruelly competitive, "capitalist" culture.

In another part of Kramer's discussion of giving Prozac to patients who, like Julia, are "too sensitive," he introduces Lucy. Lucy, a "boy-crazy" college student who once discovered her own mother's murder, suffers from heightened sensitivity to rejection. Kramer grants that Lucy's suffering is to some extent due to her in some ways impressive capacity to perceive and interpret signs that others miss. He says, however, that once Lucy took Prozac, she "moved from being confusingly perceptive—able to see people doing things that not even they knew they intended—to being perceptive in a way that allowed a less painful interaction with friends and strangers" (105).

Again, it would be at best foolish to underestimate or ignore the pain some people experience as a result of perceiving all too well. But Kramer himself worries aloud about the price we are paying to ameliorate that pain. He acknowledges that "the slight blandness apparent in some cheerful, formerly sensitive patients may reflect [a] loss of subtlety" (104).

Why worry about some people becoming less sensitive to slights? For one thing, the more we use Prozac to build up our resistance to slights, the more we can expect such slights to proliferate. That is, the faster the pace and the higher the volume of our culture, the more likely slights become. The more slights, the more we need relief. The more relief we get from a drug like Prozac, the higher our tolerance becomes. The higher our tolerance, the more likely the proliferation of such slights. All that changes are the magnitude of the stress and the dose we need for relief.

In addition to the general worry that using Prozac to reduce suffering inadvertently produces more suffering, there is the more specific worry that that suffering will fall disproportionately on those unlucky enough to have been born with personality types that currently are not valorized. As more and more people take drugs like Prozac in order to live up to the assertive, resilient, cheerful personality type, what will it be like to remain too serious, too subtle, or too sensitive when the technological option to change is available and relatively cheap? Will people who choose to remain different be made to feel like women who bear children with Down syndrome sometimes are made to feel? "Well, in the old days we would have pitied you for having a child who is different. But now? You could have gotten the amnio and you chose not to. Shame on you for messing up your life and that child's." It may be okay to be different if you never had the chance to purchase being normal. But it certainly is not okay to be different if you passed on the purchase.

As I suggested above, Kramer himself puts the worry about valorizing particular personality types front and center. Late in the book, he tries still another way to assuage that worry: by simply predicting that it probably will not happen. To the concern that the more people use drugs like Prozac to live up to current conceptions of the desirable personality type, the more others will feel pressure to do the same, he responds, "Such an outcome would clearly be bad, but it also seems unlikely, not least because of our society's aversion to prescribed medication—our 'pharmacological Calvinism'" (274). He is arguing that because so many Americans share the conviction that "if a drug makes you feel good, it must be bad," it is not reasonable to worry about the prospect of lots of Americans availing themselves of drugs just to enhance their performance and their approximation of currently fashionable personality types. Perhaps in 1993, when Kramer wrote his book, pharmacological Calvinism was alive and well. Today, however, in the land of multibillion-dollar drug sales, it is hard to find much evidence that that beast is any longer on the prowl.

Late in the book, in response to the worry that drugs like Prozac are going to produce more of the same, Kramer returns to a version of the cultural-relativism-is-nice-but-individuals-are-suffering approach mentioned earlier. Again, he writes extensively about the fact that we live in a society that values cheerfulness, resilience, and assertiveness. He knows it could be otherwise, but he constantly reminds us that it is not. We should, he suggests, accept what is. As he puts it, the expectations of our society "leave certain people difficult options: they can suffer, or they can change" (275). Nowhere in the book does he explore the possibility that instead of changing those persons who do not meet dominant expectations, we might change those expectations and the society that produces them.

Calling for society to change—and allowing individuals to suffer because they do not live up to currently fashionable conceptions of the self—can of course sound naive or cruel or both. But hoping as he does that in the end Prozac will be as good for producing rebellion as for producing conformity is, I think, at best naive.

Earlier I mentioned that Kramer holds up Woody Allen's Dr. Yang as his ideal doctor of the future: someone who uses a delicate balance of drugs and words to facilitate his patient's quest to create an authentic self and life, according to her own lights. In one respect, Dr. Yang's patient, Alice, undergoes a transformation that beautifully embodies Kramer's vision of Prozac as "a feminist drug" of empowerment and liberation. Alice does wake up to and leave the oppressive circumstances of her family and social life on the Upper East Side.

In another respect, however, Alice's transformation reminds us of what is troubling about the transformations Kramer's patients undergo. Different from Kramer's patients, whose self-transformations result in increased adaptation and/or accommodation to the dominant culture, Alice rejects that culture. As Kramer seems to forget when he presents her at the end of his book, Alice leaves the Upper East Side to work with Mother Theresa in Calcutta. She gives up her life of unfettered consumption and commits herself to a life of poverty and charity. Dr. Yang's cure allows Alice to experience the very sort of "seriousness, sensitivity, and subtlety" that Prozac can diminish.

We should, I think, be deeply skeptical about the possibility of having it both ways. We should not both affirm the proliferation of a drug that in important respects facilitates accommodation to dominant ways of being and insist that, well, that is really not so worrisome because the same drug *could* be used for resistance. Please understand: I believe that thoughtful people do and will prescribe and take drugs that aim to remedy forms of unhappiness that fall short of clinical depression. But we need to face squarely the fact that in doing so, we sometimes will be reinforcing a cultural frame that allows for narrower and narrower conceptions of authentic selves and life projects.

The vision of Prozac as a morally neutral tool that can facilitate the discovery and/or creation of our authentic selves is what relieves Kramer's anxiety. Yet no one has taught more brilliantly than he that this technology is in important respects not "morally neutral." No one has taught better than he the respect in which by listening to Prozac we have come to new understandings of what it is to be an authentic self. No one has taught more carefully than he how that understanding is shaping the kinds of life projects we think are worth pursuing and which are not. We can at once eschew the cure he offers and be grateful for the anxiety he so eloquently articulates.

NOTES

1. Peter D. Kramer, *Listening to Prozac* (New York: Viking, 1993). Further citations of this source will be indicated by page numbers in parentheses in the text.

2. See David DeGrazia's essay in this volume.

3. Peter D. Kramer, "The Valorization of Sadness: Alienation and the Melancholic Temperament," *Hastings Center Report* 30, no. 2 (2000): 15.

4. James Edwards's essay in this volume. For a nice overview of the debate, see also Bruce Jennings, "Technology and the Genetic Imaginary: Prenatal Testing and the Construction of Disability," in *Prenatal Testing and Disability Rights*, ed. Erik Parens and Adrienne Asch (Washington, D.C.: Georgetown University Press, 2000).

DAVID DeGRAZIA

Prozac, Enhancement, and Self-Creation

Marina's history was notable for significant childhood neglect. After her parents split up when Marina was four, her father became distant and mostly uninvolved. Her mother, meanwhile, suffered from depression and a borderline case of alcoholism; while involved in Marina's day-to-day life, she was inconsistently available on an emotional level. Because Marina was the oldest child and apparently "had her shit together," she was often called upon to help out with her younger sister and two brothers, who had a variety of problems ranging from depression to juvenile delinquency to significant obsessive-compulsive traits. (Family demands for her advice and assistance persisted into adulthood.) Due to the distraction of other family members' more dramatic struggles, many of Marina's own needs were never met. However nurturing this "parentified" child was, she never felt nurtured.

Although by her own account she had a troubled adolescence—doing less well than she wanted in school, flirting with drug use and reckless sexual encounters—she managed to get accepted to a good university. Settling down considerably, she excelled in college and got into a top MBA program, in which she continued her academic success. Throughout this period, her primary source of emotional sustenance came from several close friendships. Although these relationships were generally strong, Marina sometimes bristled from what she perceived to be put-downs and betrayals by those she held dear. Coming to understand how her overreaching family oppressed her, she established some reasonable boundaries with her mother and siblings, an achievement made easier by living in a different city. But her romantic life she considered a failure. Her intense work ethic afforded little time for dating, and the men she wound up with tended to be distant, rejecting, and sometimes emotionally abusive.

Throughout her life, Marina has been somewhat obsessional. She has been disturbed by thoughts about death since adolescence, being overly concerned with the possibility of tragedy befalling her or her family. These thoughts occur fleetingly and do not disrupt her functioning. For many years, her recurring sexual fantasies have featured powerful older men. She is troubled and disgusted with herself when these fantasies drive her to consume late-night hours pursuing the halfhearted titillation of sex-oriented Internet chat rooms.

As she approaches age thirty, Marina appears successful in nearly everyone's estimation: She is a well-paid manager for a large computer company, she has close friends, and she has several pastimes that she genuinely enjoys (especially bicycling and guitar playing). Yet Marina finds herself brooding and pensive, wondering about her life and its direction. She seeks out a psychiatric consultation, which takes place over four sessions, and accepts the psychiatrist's conclusion that she has no diagnosable disorder. When he suggests that psychotherapy might nevertheless be of help to her, she balks at the prospect of paying for many sessions out of pocket (since her health maintenance organization will not cover them). Still, she wants changes. At work she feels overly tentative, unsure, and too prone to worrying about possible errors. In her social life she hates how she endlessly interprets the latest transactions with friends, and she dislikes the way she is attracted to men who are bad for her but is too afraid to pursue those of more promising character. Additionally, she feels alienated by her obsessional thoughts, considering them ridiculous and bothersome, even if not significantly harmful.

After extended periods of introspection, fueled by her impending birthday and the discussions that took place in the psychiatric consultation, Marina decides that she wants to become more outgoing, confident, and decisive professionally; less prone to feelings of being socially excluded, slighted, or unworthy of a good partner; and less obsessional generally. She calls the psychiatrist who provided the consultation, whom she likes, and explains that she has heard that Prozac sometimes produces transformations like the ones she seeks—and more quickly and less expensively than one could expect from therapy. Marina requests a prescription for Prozac.

Is Marina's request morally problematic? Should a psychiatrist refuse to prescribe Prozac in a situation like this one? What may give us most pause about her request is that she wants to use a medication to change her personality and become a different sort of person. Is either the goal of major self-transformation or the means of using a prescription drug morally problematic? If so, why?

In a highly insightful set of reflections on Prozac, Carl Elliott tries to capture what would trouble many people about its use in a case like Marina's, in which personality change is among the goals.[1] In recent centuries, according to Elliott, authenticity—being true to oneself—has emerged as a widely shared value, one that is connected with people's sense of identity and what it is to live a meaningful life. From this modern perspective that values authenticity, he suggests, it may seem that deliberately changing one's personality through use of Prozac is inauthentic, resulting in a personality and life that are not really one's own. From this perspective, it "would be worrying if Prozac altered my personality, even if it gave me a better personality, simply because it isn't my personality"; after all, "What could seem less authentic, at least on the surface, than changing your personality with an antidepressant?"[2] I will counter that such a transformation can be a perfectly authentic piece of what I will call self-creation.

To focus the issue, let us examine cases of personality change via Prozac that are uncontroversially examples of enhancement. This term has been helpfully defined in bioethics as "interventions designed to improve human form or functioning beyond what is necessary to sustain or restore good health."[3] Often, enhancements are understood as interventions to produce improvements in human form or function that do not respond to genuine medical needs (where the latter are defined in terms of disease, normal functioning, or prevailing medical ideology). But sometimes enhancements are picked out by the nature of their means. Some means of self-improvement, such as exercise or education, are considered natural, virtuous, or otherwise admirable. By contrast, means that are perceived as artificial, as involving corrosive shortcuts, or as perverting medicine are often thought to render the intended self-improvement morally suspect (as with steroid use to improve performance in track).[4]

Marina's intended use of Prozac would implicate the concept of enhancement, both because she is not mentally ill and because many would perceive Prozac use as an artificial shortcut that perverts the medical enterprise. Thus her case, and those at issue in this essay, are instances of what Peter Kramer calls "cosmetic psychopharmacology" in his landmark book *Listening to Prozac*.[5] Kramer uses the term to describe Prozac's effect on patients who are not really ill and who become "better than well": more energetic, confident, and socially attractive. It is worth noting that, to varying degrees, certain other drugs—such as Ritalin for increasing attention span, other "smart drugs," propranolol for reducing normal anxiety and enhancing musical performance, and the "happy pill" ginseng—raise at least some of the issues associated with cosmetic psychopharmacology.[6] But this essay will concentrate on Prozac, which apparently produces the most extensive transformations of personality and therefore presents the issues of enhancement and self-creation in the clearest light.

The modern sensibility Elliott characterizes suggests that it would be inauthentic, and therefore morally problematic, for Marina to use Prozac for the purpose of changing her personality; indeed, if the drug had its intended effect, the resulting personality would not really be hers. However intuitively appealing this reasoning may be, it is undermined by its misleading image of the self as "given," static, or something there to be discovered. I hold that one can be true to oneself even as one deliberately transforms—to some extent creating—oneself. The remainder of this essay pursues these claims in greater detail.

AUTHENTICITY

Elliott's remarks about Prozac and authenticity occur within a broader discussion of values pervading contemporary American culture, and much of this discussion takes us beyond the issues considered here. What interests me is his take on the ethics of authenticity, to which he ascribes two leading ideas (without necessarily endorsing these ideas), and the possible implications of this approach for people like Marina.[7]

The first leading idea of the ethics of authenticity, Elliott states, is that life is a project whose meaning depends on how we live and for which we are largely responsible. I agree with this claim. The second main idea, according to Elliott, may be broken into two parts. First, figuring out how one should live requires introspection, because there is no unique external standard for living meaningfully. Here again I agree (while noting the role introspection plays in Marina's growth). Second, one has to discover and be true to oneself in order to live an authentic life. To the extent that this assertion suggests that the self is "given," a preexisting reality that might be discovered and to which one's actions should conform ("be true"), it strikes me as highly problematic for neglecting the possibilities of self-creation.

I turn now to my reasons for rejecting this assertion and to the image of the self on which it depends.

The ideas of authenticity, of being true to oneself, and of self-creation provoke concerns pertaining to personal identity. But what sense of identity is at issue? One interpretation of the term, which has been analyzed with insight by John Locke and with virtuosity by Derek Parfit and kindred contemporary philosophers, is that of numerical identity over time.[8] A thing at one time is numerically identical with something at another time if both are literally the same object, which is consistent with the object's undergoing qualitative change over time. In this sense of identity, the problem of personal identity is to specify the conditions that must be satisfied for a person to continue to exist through time. While this concept of personal identity raises interesting issues concerning the definition of death, the authority of advance directives in cases of severe dementia, and other practical problems, it is not the sense of identity that is central to the present discussion.[9]

The sense of personal identity at the heart of issues of authenticity and self-creation is that connected with our self-conceptions, what we consider most important to who we are, and our self-told narratives about our own lives. Your inner story allows you to get your bearings when you act, especially when confronting difficult or momentous decisions.[10] It is what comes apart when a person has an identity crisis, which leaves her or him, in an important sense, wondering who she or he is.[11] In this sense of identity, one could become a different person by undergoing a major change of outlook and values. And this is the notion Kramer has in mind when he describes the transforming effects of Prozac: Someone on Prozac might acquire a new sense of self—or identity—and strike others as having become "a new person."

All of this suggests that the self (sense of self, identity) can change over time. Indeed, the feeling that a self might undergo too much change may underlie some of the common discomfort with cosmetic psychopharmacology. But how malleable is the self, and to what extent can one actively change oneself? It is important to have a tenable view on these issues before considering possibilities for self-creation and the notion of whether self-creation via Prozac can be authentic.

One possible view envisions the self as completely given, though one may have to dig—with reflection, therapy, or the like—to discover its shape and true colors. Though one can find the self, one cannot actively change it; any change in the self over time is due to forces outside one's agency. One version of this view takes the self or "inner core" (self-defining, individual values) to be entirely constructed by society.[12]

Another possible position, essentially the opposite, takes the self to be as amorphous and malleable as Silly Putty. In Jean-Paul Sartre's view, for example, we human beings are thrown into the world without any determinate nature. What we choose determines what we are, so we are completely responsible for what we become. With nothing except ourselves determining our actions and identities, we shoulder the burden of radical freedom. Thus we may shape ourselves into one form one day without limiting what we can shape ourselves into the next day. In this view, one is entirely self-creating, leaving no room for discovering anything about oneself, except perhaps what one freely chooses to be.[13]

These two extreme views about self-malleability strike me as highly implausible, but I will not advance philosophical arguments in an effort to refute them. Readers are simply invited to reflect on their experiences of themselves and familiar others, to determine whether the following claims ring true.

Our efforts at self-improvement, however fumbling and imperfect, suggest that we can reshape ourselves to some extent and that at least some of the reshaping is due to our own efforts. For example, we may try with some success to become more disciplined—or perhaps less disciplined, for the workaholics and perfectionists among us. We may work at being more generous or more patient or more willing to stand up to authority, and sometimes we may succeed. We may aspire to orient ourselves more toward a relationship—or less toward any relationship if we need to be more independent. When we accomplish change in ourselves, it does not seem that the catalyst of this change is entirely independent of our agency (as it would be if the impetus were simply social forces, human nature, or one's genetic makeup). But if human phenomenology suggests a capacity for self-change through our agency, it does not suggest an unlimited capacity. Addicts and persons with obsessive-compulsive disorder, for example, know that their will is not the only force driving their actions. And all of us are frequently reminded that there are limits to what our efforts can accomplish in changing our characters and behavior, just as there are limits to what our bodies can achieve in sports. The best metaphor I have come across for capturing the moderate view recommended here pictures the self as wood that can be sculpted, "respecting the constraints of natural shape and grain."[14]

DAVID DEGRAZIA

This moderate view allows for the possibility of some degree of self-creation. Jonathan Glover, whose work on this topic has greatly influenced my thinking, defines self-creation as "consciously shaping our own characteristics."[15] Specifying the concept a bit for present purposes, I understand it to involve consciously and deliberately shaping one's own personality, character, or life direction in nontrivial ways.

Assuming, as the above reflections suggest, that such self-shaping is possible, it should be understood as one crucial process that determines what we and our lives become. The possibilities for self-creation are limited by its enmeshment with other crucial processes and factors.[16] One of these is the genetically determined cycle of life, which we are not free to escape: the neediness of infancy and childhood, the relative turbulence of adolescence, the gradual loss of certain physical powers in advanced age, and so on. Other crucial factors concern the tools we are given to work with, especially our particular genetic endowment and the quality of our early environment. A final important consideration—which might easily be overlooked—is the set of unexpected, seemingly random yet momentous consequences of the things we choose. To offer an autobiographical example, I once decided, somewhat reluctantly and without great interest, to attend a Halloween party, where I happened to meet the woman who later became my wife and the mother of my child. While self-creation is possible, the range of possibilities open to an individual is at once expanded and limited by other major processes and factors that shape our lives.

People who are engaged in self-creation seek to change themselves. Marina, for example, wants to change her personality. While she has been tentative, socially a bit mistrustful, and somewhat obsessive for as long as she can remember, she would like to be free of these personality traits. But this raises a conceptual issue: If Marina loses these characteristics, will the resulting person really be Marina?[17]

The modern conception of authenticity, as Elliott characterizes it, suggests at least the possibility of a negative answer. But I think a negative answer here is profoundly mistaken—and not just because of the associated image of a static self. For, again, what is identity in the relevant sense all about? It is about one's self-conception, what a person considers most important to who she or he is, her or his self-told inner story. That means that it is ultimately up to Marina to determine what counts as Marina and what counts as not-Marina; the story is hers to write (within reality constraints set by the factors and processes described earlier). And she wants to get rid of the traits in question, if she can. In general, whether certain personality traits are definitive of someone depends on whether that individual identifies with them — that is, whether she or he owns them (pun intended) autonomously. An example will help make the point.

Imagine two people, Nina and Xena, both of whom are inveterate, addicted cigarette smokers. Both spend a lot of money on cigarettes, both find the habit very inconvenient at times (like when they run low late at night and have to bother friends for rides to the nearest convenience store), and both are unsure they could muster the willpower to quit if they tried. Is being a smoker part of their respective identities? In my view, that depends on further detail.

Suppose that they have different attitudes toward their addiction. Nina finds it alien and out of character (not-her) and wishes she had never smoked that first cigarette. Xena, meanwhile, delights in being contrarian and knows that smoking and addiction generally are contrary to (what most people consider) good sense. While, in a way, her addiction makes her unfree not to smoke — she just has to light up periodically — Xena is autonomously a smoker, precisely because she identifies with smoking along with its delightfully contrarian associations.[18] So while both women are smokers, being a smoker is part of Xena's identity but not part of Nina's, and the difference lies in their distinct value systems.

This consequence should not be surprising, since who we are has everything to do with what we value. And what we value largely determines our projects of self-creation. Thus, if Marina is able to rid herself of traits with which she does not identify and decides that the "real Marina" does not have those traits, no one is in a position to contradict her.

What legitimate basis might there be, then, for the idea that it would be inauthentic for Marina to change her personality? Do the means of chosen personality change — using Prozac — matter here? Some would answer affirmatively, contending that these means represent an unnatural or artificial shortcut to self-improvement. But such a view, however intuitively appealing, appears prejudicial when carefully examined.

Consider a path to desired self-change that would be regarded as natural and admirably laborious (not to mention clearly within the bounds of accepted psychiatric practice): psychotherapy. Successful psychotherapy sometimes produces a shift in personality that the patient considers an improvement.[19] Now suppose Marina wanted to change her personality through the long, hard work of therapy. If she

DAVID DEGRAZIA

were willing to pay for it, I can imagine no reasonable objection to her enhancement project ("cosmetic psychotherapy," we might call it, keeping in mind that she is not genuinely ill). So I take it that therapy is an authentic and otherwise legitimate way of facilitating self-creation, even where enhancement is the goal.

The question is, Why should the supposedly unnatural shortcut of Prozac use make any significant difference to the authenticity of Marina's self-creation project? It seems irrelevant that it is unnatural—that it works directly on her biochemistry, rather than indirectly on her biochemistry, as therapy often does (by affecting the patient's emotional life). The shortcut would still be authentic because Marina's values and self-conception are the basis for the chosen means. To be sure, in some contexts certain unnatural means are contrary to the spirit of a competition (e.g., steroid use in track and field) and in that sense constitute cheating—perhaps even a type of inauthenticity. But Marina's situation is nothing like this; she is simply trying to live her life. Moreover, that her plan involves a shortcut might, in some ways, make it admirable from a prudential standpoint. After all, it is her time and money that will be consumed here.

Therapy may offer some advantages to a patient that Prozac does not offer (as discussed later). But if Marina does not find those advantages to offset the efficiency she hopes to find in Prozac, it is hard to see the basis for paternalistically judging that her values and self-conception are not authoritative for her own life—not only for what is good in her life (best interests) but also for what constitutes her life (authenticity). I therefore conclude that Prozac, no less than psychotherapy, can be an authentic part of a project of self-creation.

REMAINING WORRIES

If the preceding arguments have been sound, they show that using Prozac can be an authentic part of a self-creation project, even in cases that involve enhancement. This conclusion seems generalizable to other instances of cosmetic psychopharmacology—assuming, as with Marina, that an adult with decision-making capacity is deciding only for herself, since decisions for children and incapacitated adults raise special issues.[20] But even if the charge of inauthenticity is wrongheaded, it does not follow that cosmetic psychopharmacology is ethically justified or wise. While this essay has focused on the issues of authenticity and self-creation in relation to Prozac, here I will enumerate some substantial ethical concerns that remain about cosmetic psychopharmacology for capable adults like Marina, concerns that go well beyond those raised by Elliott's remarks. In the end, I do not think these concerns demonstrate that Marina's psychiatrist should refrain from prescribing Prozac for her, or that Marina should exclude Prozac from her project of self-creation. But, for reasons of space, I will only gesture in the direction of an adequate reply to each concern en passant.

One concern is that Prozac, and other pharmaceuticals that could be used for enhancement purposes, are not available to all who might want and stand to benefit from them.[21] Approximately 40 million Americans lack health insurance; many others are insured by plans that do not cover prescriptions for psychiatric medications or provide coverage only when one has a diagnosable illness. Of course, the relatively wealthy can still opt to pay out of pocket. But the overall picture is one in which cosmetic psychopharmacology is likely to benefit mainly those who are relatively well-off and otherwise advantaged. Thus, by exacerbating existing gaps between the haves and have-nots in our society, cosmetic psychopharmacology raises issues of social and economic fairness.

These concerns about unfairness are legitimate. But the unfairness is more sensibly located in our entire economic system—including our system of health care finance (which promotes the interests of the private insurance industry at nearly everyone's expense)—than in Marina's or her psychiatrist's choices. In my view, they and everyone else should fight for greater justice in the distribution of income, wealth, and health care access, but doing so is compatible with Marina's use of Prozac. Note, by the way, that if Marina is right that taking Prozac would cost less than psychotherapy undertaken for the same goals, her project is less criticizable on the present grounds than therapy would be, since the more expensive approach would be available to even fewer people.

Another worry is that cosmetic psychopharmacology tends to promote some very troubling cultural values. Part of what drives Marina's interest, for example, is her desire to be more efficient at work and her longing for a more attractive personality. Considering that she is already professionally successful and has good friendships, one might perceive her desire for self-improvement to reflect our culture's disturbing tendency to valorize hypercompetitiveness and "designer" personalities. Thus her plan and her psychiatrist's involvement (if he goes along) raise the issue of complicity with suspect social norms.[22]

DAVID DeGRAZIA

While I agree that our society overvalues competitiveness and other yuppie-oriented qualities, it seems to me that reasonable people could disagree with this judgment. In any case, the concern should be located in our broader culture (which is arguably too deferential to a capitalist mindset), not placed in the laps of Marina and her psychiatrist. If there is a responsibility to change the culture, it is everyone's responsibility and should not be arbitrarily imposed on particular individuals by interfering with their self-regarding projects.

Some critics also feel that widespread use of Prozac and similar drugs, unlike psychotherapy, promotes biopsychiatry's agenda of reducing emotional and personal struggles to mechanistic terms—as if these struggles were just another form of pain to be treated with a new pill.[23] Primarily benefiting drug companies and biopsychiatric researchers, according to critics, this agenda threatens our self-conceptions as reasonable agents.

In response, people might not be equally troubled by the possibility that Prozac use supports biopsychiatry's agendas. In any event, Marina and her psychiatrist have no obligation to promote the symbolism of human beings as reasonable agents. We are such agents, but we are also feeling creatures; self-esteem problems, suspiciousness, and compulsiveness are connected with our agency, but they are also closely connected to unpleasant feelings, which Prozac may help to alleviate. Besides, even if Prozac use has some mechanistic associations, Marina's plan for changing herself and her life direction is a powerful expression of her own agency.

Several other concerns can be stated more briefly. One is that cosmetic psychopharmacology can encourage social quietism. The idea is that drug-induced complacency may be favored over active struggle to change the social conditions (e.g., dangerous work environments or poor social supports for working parents) that contribute to patients' discontent, with the result that these social problems are left untouched.[24] In response, while there may be some risk of social quietism, the risk attaches to all use of mood-improving drugs (not just to cases of cosmetic psychopharmacology), to mainstream religions, and to many other clearly acceptable practices and institutions that brighten our outlooks.

Another criticism concerns those who pursue cosmetic psychopharmacology for competitive reasons, such as wanting to become more confident businesspersons. If nearly everyone in a particular competitive environment makes the same choice, the result will be self-defeating to all: Increased expense and other personal costs of taking the drug and no advantage over others (just as most law school applicants take an LSAT prep course without gaining a competitive advantage).[25] Meanwhile, those who would prefer not to take the drug may feel social pressure and possibly coercion to do so out of fear of falling too far behind.[26] At least with respect to Prozac, the concerns about self-defeating drug enhancements and about excessive social pressure are rather speculative, because presently we are far from such a scenario.[27] What to do if and when it arrives, however, is not at all obvious (just as there is no obvious solution to the problem concerning the LSAT prep course). But the mere possibility of such a scenario does not, in my view, cast significant moral doubt on Marina's enhancement project.

Finally, we should not ignore whatever risks are associated with the drug in question, especially since some risks may remain unknown while others may be hard to discern accurately amid the glitter of celebrated benefits. This concern highlights the importance of an informed consent process that includes a responsible, balanced, and thorough discussion of risks; it does not justify paternalistically precluding use of the drugs in question.

CONCLUDING REFLECTIONS

While there are some substantial ethical concerns about cosmetic psychopharmacology, even in the case of capable adults, these concerns do not suggest that Marina's plan of Prozac use is illegitimate or that her psychiatrist should refuse to write a prescription. (Of course, if any of these ethical concerns so troubles her psychiatrist that he feels he cannot in good conscience take part in her plan, he has no obligation to do so.) But even if my overall assessment of these ethical concerns were mistaken, this would not undermine the major goal of this essay: to show that a transformation via cosmetic psychopharmacology can be a perfectly authentic piece of self-creation, so that the resulting personality and life are very much one's one. One can identify with certain traits, authentically pursue them, and change oneself— while maintaining one's identity—within a project of self-creation. Indeed, as the tone of this essay may have revealed, I believe such self-transformation can be quite admirable.

At the same time, the wisest path toward desired self-creation may often include the slow, arduous road of psychotherapy, despite its considerable costs. For those who are willing to work and confront some unpleasantness about themselves or their lives, and who possess at least ordinary introspective capacities, psychotherapy offers insights that are generally not available from other sources or activities. Moreover, any enhancements of personality, character, or life plans that result from this vigorous work stand a decent chance of lasting. Meanwhile, those who go the route of cosmetic psychopharmacology may need to take drugs indefinitely to maintain whatever desired changes are achieved. (Perhaps, then, we should question the assumption that therapy is more expensive, at least in the long run.)

If Marina were my friend or family member, I would urge her to take the possibility of extended therapy very seriously. I might even try to make the case that its likely benefits more than offset its added costs. But the ultimate values that count here, the ones that must be translated into benefits and costs of various weights, are Marina's. So if she perceives her options with eyes wide open, she should be allowed to select that which is best for her (assuming a psychiatrist is willing to help). It is, after all, her life—and her identity.

NOTES

1. Carl Elliott, "The Tyranny of Happiness: Ethics and Cosmetic Psychopharmacology," in *Enhancing Human Traits: Ethical and Social Implications*, ed. Erik Parens (Washington, D.C.: Georgetown University Press, 1998).

2. Ibid., 182, 186. Erik Parens, who edited the excellent anthology that contains Elliott's article, seems to concur with this sentiment. Thus Parens speaks of "appreciating that drugs like Prozac are good at promoting self-fulfillment *as opposed to authenticity*" ("Is Better Always Good? The Enhancement Project," in Parens, *Enhancing Human Traits*, 23, my emphasis).

3. Eric T. Juengst, "What Does Enhancement Mean?," in Parens, *Enhancing Human Traits*, 29.

4. For a detailed discussion of these different senses of enhancement, see ibid.

5. Peter D. Kramer, *Listening to Prozac* (New York: Viking, 1993).

6. See, e.g., Lawrence H. Diller, "The Run on Ritalin: Attention Deficit Disorder and Stimulant Treatment in the 1990s," *Hastings Center Report* 26, no. 2 (1996): 12–18; Claudia Mills, "One Pill Makes You Smarter: An Ethical Appraisal of the Rise of Ritalin," *Report from the Institute for Philosophy and Public Policy* 18, no. 4 (1998): 13–17; Peter J. Whitehouse et al., "Enhancing Cognition in the Intellectually Intact," *Hastings Center Report* 27, no. 3 (1997): 14–22; Jacquelyn Slomka, "Playing with Propranolol," *Hastings Center Report* 22, no. 4 (1992): 13–17; and Jonathan Glover, *What Sort of People Should There Be?* (London: Penguin, 1984), 71–72 (on ginseng).

7. Elliott, "Tyranny of Happiness," 181–82. Elliott cites Charles Taylor, Lionel Trilling, and Michael Walzer.

8. See, e.g., John Locke, *Essay Concerning Human Understanding*, 2nd ed. (1694), bk. 2, chap. 27; H. P. Grice, "Personal Identity," *Mind* 50 (1941): 330–50; Sidney Shoemaker, "Persons and Their Pasts," *American Philosophical Quarterly* 7 (1970): 269–85; John Perry, "Can the Self Divide?," *Journal of Philosophy* 69 (1972): 463–88; Derek Parfit, *Reasons and Persons* (Oxford: Clarendon, 1984); Harold W. Noonan, *Personal Identity* (London: Routledge, 1989); Raymond Martin, *Self-Concern* (Cambridge: Cambridge University Press, 1998); Lynn Rudder Baker, *Persons and Bodies* (Cambridge: Cambridge University Press, 2000); and Jeff McMahan, *The Ethics of Killing* (New York: Oxford University Press, 2002), chap. 1.

9. See my "Identity, Killing, and the Boundaries of Our Existence," *Philosophy and Public Affairs* 31, no. 4 (2003): 413–43. These themes along with those examined in the present essay are explored in greater detail in *Human Identity and Bioethics* (Cambridge University Press, forthcoming).

10. Jonathan Glover, *I: The Philosophy and Psychology of Personal Identity* (London: Penguin, 1988), 152.

11. Marya Schechtman emphasizes this point in what may be the strongest theoretical exploration of this sense of personal identity; see *The Constitution of Selves* (Ithaca, N.Y.: Cornell University Press, 1961), esp. pt. 2.

12. This position is helpfully explored and criticized in Glover, *I*, chap. 17.

13. Jean-Paul Sartre, *Being and Nothingness*, trans. H. E. Barnes (New York: Philosophical Library, 1956).

14. Glover, *I*, 136.

15. Ibid., 131.

16. Here again I largely follow Glover (ibid., 138), who seems to reflect enlightened common sense.

17. Kramer raises this conceptual issue in the case of his own patients (see, e.g., *Listening to Prozac*, 18–19).

18. I explore the distinction between liberty (freedom) of action and autonomy in "Autonomous Action and Autonomy-Subverting Psychiatric Conditions," *Journal of Medicine and Philosophy* 19 (1994): 279–97. My analysis is influenced by Harry Frankfurt, "Freedom of the Will and the Concept of a Person," *Journal of Philosophy* 68 (1971): 829–39; Gerald Dworkin, "Autonomy and Behavior Control," *Hastings Center Report* 6 (1976): 23–28; and John Christman, "Autonomy: A Defense of the Split-Level Self," *Southern Journal of Philosophy* 25 (1987): 281–93.

19. Sometimes a personality change may result from the patient's rewriting her or his inner story, since this story is about who she or he is. Cf.

Glover, *I*, 153. For a classic background work, see Sigmund Freud, *Introductory Lectures on Psychoanalysis* (1920; reprint, New York: Norton, 1960).

20. Much of the concern about Ritalin, for example, focuses on parental consent on behalf of children, sometimes in apparent conflict with their best interests. See, e.g., Diller, "Run on Ritalin," and Mills, "One Pill Makes You Smarter."

21. Dan W. Brock, "Enhancements of Human Function: Some Distinctions for Policymakers," in Parens, *Enhancing Human Traits*, 59.

22. Cf. Elliott, "Tyranny of Happiness." Regarding this problem in connection with Ritalin, see Diller, "Run on Ritalin," 17; regarding the more frightening case of prescribing for children, see Mills, "One Pill Makes You Smarter," 16–17. For an insightful discussion of complicity with suspect cultural norms, see Margaret Olivia Little, "Cosmetic Surgery, Suspect Norms, and the Ethics of Complicity," in Parens, *Enhancing Human Traits*, 162–76.

23. This viewpoint is powerfully developed in Carol Freedman, "Aspirin for the Mind? Some Ethical Worries about Psychopharmacology," in Parens, *Enhancing Human Traits*, 135–50.

24. See Elliott, "Tyranny of Happiness," 180; Glover, *What Sort of People Should There Be?*, 72–73; and Diller, "Run on Ritalin," 14–15.

25. Brock, "Enhancements of Human Function," 60.

26. See Diller, "Run on Ritalin," 16, and Slomka, "Playing with Propranolol," 15.

27. We are probably closer in the cases of Ritalin for schoolchildren and propranolol for professional musicians (see cites in preceding note). My sense is that the associated difficulties are so closely tied to the features of a particular drug and the social context in which it is used that we cannot profitably generalize from a viable solution for one drug to cosmetic psychopharmacology in general.

PETER D. KRAMER

The Valorization of Sadness
Alienation and the Melancholic Temperament

At the heart of *Listening to Prozac* is a thought experiment: Imagine that we have a medication that can move a person from a normal psychological state to another normal psychological state that is more desired or better socially rewarded.[1] What are the moral consequences of that potential, the one I called cosmetic psychopharmacology?

The question would be overgeneral except that it occurs in the context of a discussion of psychic consequences of technologies. People now experience the self in the light of psychotherapeutic medications as lately they experienced it through psychoanalysis. In the thought experiment, the medication we are to imagine is rather like Prozac, and the less desired state is something like melancholy, when that term refers to a personality style rather than an illness. Melancholics are well described in literature that stretches back for centuries. They are pessimistic, self-doubting, moralistic, and obsessive. They have low energy but use that energy productively. They are creative in the arts. They are prone to depression, especially in response to social disappointments.

Listening to Prozac argues that the important action of new medications may be on the melancholic temperament as much as on depression, although the two are presumed to be related. The book's assessment of cosmetic psychopharmacology begins with the observation that for decades, psychotherapy has been the technology applied to melancholy. In this account, psychotherapy includes approaches, such as supportive or strategic therapies, in which self-understanding is not the means or end of cure—where the goal is change in affective state merely. Asking why cosmetic psychopharmacology makes us so uneasy, I did not neglect to consider the targets of treatment—in particular, claims that suffering is an indicator of the human condition, that psychic pain serves an adaptive function, and that melancholy is an element of authentic self. But since the premise of "cosmesis" is movement from normal to normal, the posttreatment as much as the pretreatment state should meet the criteria of Darwinian fitness and human completeness. Those who hope psychotherapy succeeds must be comfortable with the diminution of melancholy. For these reasons, I came to believe that a critical element in a principled objection to cosmetic psychopharmacology must involve the method of change, namely, medication, more than the goals of intervention.

To my delight moral philosophers, particularly medical ethicist Carl Elliott, have taken up this thought experiment in a series of essays distinguished by their literary appeal. These discussions are a continuation of *Listening to Prozac*, but they are also a form of backtracking, because the element that interests Elliott is cosmesis's goal. Elliott is worried about the diminution of alienation.

I hope here to use Elliott's essays to ask, as rule keeper for a certain sort of game, whether the concept of alienation successfully identifies grounds on which cosmetic psychopharmacology might be morally suspect. At the same time, I will want to reopen the issue of the legitimate goals of treatment. To preview my conclusion, my impression is that the concern over Prozac, and with imagined medications extrapolated from experience with Prozac, turns almost entirely on an aesthetic valuation of melancholy.

Elliott's central claim is that addressing alienation as a psychiatric issue is like treating Holy Communion as a dietary issue: a category mistake. Included in this claim is the understanding that alienation has a particular moral worth. Neither of these assertions strikes me as obvious. In particular, I want to say that both are thrown into doubt by a premise of our discussion, namely, that medication can lessen alienation. The nature of the technology may cause us to reassess the category, and the significance, of the target.

To begin with the question of category: Clearly *some* alienation is an aspect of mental illness; indeed, alienation is an element in schizophrenia. It is not absurd to imagine that alienation might be "psychiatric." Often Elliott equates alienation with depression, as when he paraphrases Walker Percy to this effect: "Take a look around you; it would take a moron not to be depressed."[2] The arguments Elliott makes regarding depression and alienation, as worrisome targets for pharmacology, are identical. It is not always clear whether the depression referred to is a stance or a syndrome.

As regards category, then, the question is alienation of what sort?

Elliott recognizes that alienation comes in many forms, and he describes personal, cultural, and existential alienation. But from a psychiatric point of view, the people Elliott suggests as candidates for antidepressant use are homogeneous. They are not primarily mistrustful in a way that might make us think of a paranoid alienation, nor are they socially unaware and distanced from their fellows in a way that might suggest an autistic alienation. Elliott's subjects are sad, obsessive, and questing. They worry. Their alienation is of a single sort, the sort that is an element of the melancholic personality.

When I say that the premise "medication diminishes alienation" casts its shadow on questions of category, I mean that our likely beliefs about category are susceptible to being altered by our beliefs about how that diminution occurs. We do not expect medication to work directly on the cognitive component of alienation, just as we do not imagine there is a pill for, say, atheism or chauvinism; that sort of imagining would violate the rule that the drug we have in mind is a good deal like Prozac. Presumably, our hypothetic medication tones down obsessionality, pessimism, and social anxiety, so that, secondarily, a person feels less impelled to resist the ambient culture. It alters affective aspects of personality, where affect extends to such phenomena as sense of status in social groups.

That is to say, our premise brings into play the basis of personality. If we were certain, as many midcentury psychoanalysts were, that personality is the detailed psychic encoding of a person's experience in the world, relatively fixed but responsive to insight, then the parameters for a discussion of the pharmacologic enhancement of alienation would be clearer. Equally, if we were to discover that even minor depression is in all instances caused by a virus that deforms brain anatomy, the discussion would be stable at a different point of equilibrium. The range of philosophical arguments might remain similar—one can approach character armor as a medical condition and one can define living with microbes as an expectable state of human life—but in each instance we would be more inclined to entertain particular explanations.

To clarify the interplay of target and technology: Setting aside Prozac, let us imagine that it is discovered that moderate doses of vitamin C decrease a person's sense of isolation. Would the taking of vitamins seem worrisome? The answer depends on how we "listen" to the medication. We might decide that alienation of that sort was in all probability something like a vitamin deficiency. We might even decide in retrospect that our objection to cosmesis had resulted from an

PETER D. KRAMER

aesthetic assessment of the technology employed to achieve it. That is, previously (when it was a matter of using Prozac rather than vitamins to the same end) we had objected because the technology was artificial, scientifically complex, and manufactured and advertised by a large corporation—partaking of the very qualities we believe ought to lead to alienation, on, say, a political basis. Once vitamin C's effect was discovered, we might come to believe that Prozac had, after all, been repairing medical damage to the self. Starting with the premise that medication can mitigate alienation, it is not hard to imagine evidence in light of which alienation would be most parsimoniously understood as at least in part a psychiatric issue.

I should add that as a clinician, I find the argument by category mistake suspect because, generally, category mistakes are in the opposite direction from the one that perturbs Elliott. Mental illness has too often been too narrowly understood—misunderstood as a principled response to social conditions; this error is one R. D. Laing made with regard to schizophrenia when he claimed that psychosis is a response to the absurd pressures of bourgeois family life. My own belief is that the conundrum necessarily is played out at a historical moment, ours, when the categorization of alienation remains ambiguous.

Elliott goes on to argue that alienation is circumstantially appropriate and morally valuable. Regarding personal and cultural alienation—the mismatch between particular self and the particulars of the social surroundings—Elliott writes that you might feel ill at ease among Milwaukee Rotarians. Elliott would disfavor your being offered Prozac in this instance because "some external circumstances call for alienation."

Now I hope that no one is dispensing medication as an alternative to dropping membership in the Milwaukee Rotary. But if Elliott is at some distance from the clinical moment here, he is nonetheless successful in depicting one sort of unease, that of the sensitive person stuck in a group of philistines. Walker Percy, in a passage cited by Elliott, works the same vein as regards depression: "Consider the only adults who are never depressed: chuckleheads, California surfers, and fundamentalist Christians who believe they have had a personal encounter with Jesus and are saved once and for all. Would you trade your depression to become any one of these?"[3]

These examples are amusing, but I fear that because they are all of a type, they prejudice the jury. Elliott's and Percy's comments succeed, on first reading, not because we value every instance of alienation—

any sort of fish out of any sort of water—but because of a cultural preference for the melancholic over the sanguine. Consider the alienation or depression of a hockey player (a potential future Rotarian) rooming with poets; we may not want him to resist integration. Or consider the sort of movie, common in recent years, in which a straitlaced man is thrown into the company of a wild woman and her friends; the audience's hope is that he will overcome rather than sustain his alienation from the kooky subculture.

In *Listening to Prozac*, I addressed a similar issue—alienation from what?—in regard to mourning rituals. Those who consider the American grieving period too brief and therefore alienating to the sensitive have pointed with admiration to rural Greece, where widows mourn predeceasing husbands for five years. But enforced mourning is restrictive for resilient widows; they are the alienated in a traditional culture. If alienation means a sense of incompatibility with the environment, then people of differing temperaments will be alienated in different settings. Do we honor both the sensitive and the resilient? Is it permissible for resilient Greek women to move to a society with shorter grieving periods? More to the point, if the sensitive move to rural Greece, will the consequent loss of alienation rob them of an aspect of their humanity? This sort of example might convince us that it is not personal or cultural alienation that we value, but the melancholic temperament or aspects of it, such as loyalty and sensitivity—and that we honor a sufferer in any setting, even one from which he or she is not personally or culturally alienated.

Effectively, Elliott conflates personal and cultural alienation. The notion of cultural alienation is invisibly buttressed by what I might call the Woody Allen effect. The prominently neurotic today are often political liberals, and this correlation has more or less held since the Romantic era. Soft left, hard right. But even if this conjunction is real and has an explanation (and what sort of explanation do we have in mind?), it is hardly universal. A sanguine person may be alarmed by apartheid, just as a melancholic might attribute his or her disaffection to the ending of apartheid. If Prozac induces conformity, it is to an ideal of assertiveness, but assertiveness can be in the service of social reform of the sort ordinarily understood as nonconformity or rebellion. The political effects of medicating the disaffected will be various.

Politics aside, we may find we have an aesthetic preference for neurosis. The melancholic temperament is the artistic temperament. Even if hearty Apollonian artists exist—Lionel Trilling and Edmund Wilson debated the point—they are less appealing than the wounded Dionysian variety.[4] The cluster of personality traits arising from the melancholic temperament (pessimism, perfectionism, sensitivity, and the rest) overlaps so strongly with our image of the intellectual that we may have difficulty crediting thinkers who are differently constituted. The pervasiveness of this valuation came home to me in the course of my writing an essay about psychologist Carl Rogers; Rogers met all the criteria for intellectuality save one, pessimism, and on that ground was dismissed as a lightweight.[5]

Thus concern over personal or cultural alienation comes to seem the valuation of one sort of normal person (the melancholic) over another (the sanguine). And just how far would a moralist go in this preference for alienation? Are those 25 percent of humans who lack the purported "Woody Allen gene" morally defective? If so, we might logically favor a medication that makes them more ill at ease. It seems less a matter of mistrusting pharmacology than of valuing melancholy.

Elliott's third category is existential alienation—"questioning the very terms on which a life is built," an unease such as one might suffer even on a desert island or, as Robert Coles might put it, under any moon. Here we seem to be getting to the heart of the matter, alienation that has nothing to do with distance from a particular social surround.

We could perhaps obviate this consideration by arguing that if existential alienation is neither personal nor cultural, it should be part of being human, for all people in all times. If normal life is a project, then change qualifies as cosmetic only when life remains a project. Even for "good responders" to medication, existence remains hedged by death, chance, unfairness, and absurdity.

But empirically we know that angst grabs different people differently. Some people are more constantly aware of the universal existential condition. But what is it to be aware in this sense? Even existential alienation might be intertwined with temperament. Elliott leans toward that recognition when he writes, "Alienation of any type might go together with depression, of course, but I suspect that the two do not necessarily go hand in hand." But that is the question at issue: To what extent is affect, such as anxiety or depression, constitutive of existential alienation? To put the matter differently: If, medicated, one retains an intellectual unease but with diminished emotional discomfort, does being in that state constitute existential alienation?

Imagine one of Walker Percy's famously alienated characters, say, a commuter. He might feel bad for two reasons: because life is imperfect and because he is predisposed to feel worse than others do in response to that imperfection. If he experiences relief via medication, he might come to understand which was which, his dysthymia versus the alienation common to all humans. As a diagnostician, medication is imperfect, but neither is it simply dismissible. On a quest for authenticity, we must be open to discoveries of this sort—that what seemed carefully developed self was arbitrary, biologically based idiosyncrasy.

Elliott resists this sort of reframing when he asserts that "there is no difference between the commuter who feels bad without knowing why and the same commuter reading a copy of DSM-IV."[6] But that is because Elliott mistrusts the manual. Finding his condition delineated there, the commuter might decide he had formerly made a category mistake, just as, finding himself in a Walker Percy novel, a diagnosed depressive might draw a conclusion in the reverse direction. I once treated a dysthymic patient whose former psychiatrist had commanded her to "put away your Sylvia Plath!" Whether poetry or medication (or manual-reading) is a better means to self-discovery is in part an empirical question; a combination might prove optimal.

Another thought experiment: Imagine we have defined possible elements of existential alienation, such as spleen, anomie, angst, accedia, vertigo, malaise, emptiness, and the like. Now we give a medication for depression and find that some factors disappear and others remain, so that a hypothetical subject is no longer vertiginous but remains anomic. Would we have defined "core" alienation? Dissected the existential? Well, perhaps not—not if alienation's connection to minor depression is especially intimate. The problem of melancholic temperament cannot be made to disappear, not even by our framing the conundrum in terms of respect for existential alienation. Elliott's worry is precisely that if a medication replaces pessimism with optimism, anxiety with assertiveness, and diffidence with gregariousness, it will have robbed us of a tendency to remain at a critical distance from our own existence. The affective stance is what is of value, worrying the same old bone, as Percy puts it—not mere awareness of distance but anxiety over it.

I have come to believe that much of the discussion of cosmetic psychopharmacology is not about pharmacology at all—that is to say, not about the technology. Rather, cosmetic pharmacology is a stand-in for worries over threats to melancholy. That psychotherapy caused less worry may speak to our lack of confidence in its efficacy.

We do, as a culture, value melancholy. Some months ago, I attended an exhibition of the paintings of "the young Picasso." Seeing the early canvases, I thought, "Here is a marvelous technician." I turned a cor-

PETER D. KRAMER

ner to confront the works of the Blue Period, Picasso's response to the suicide of his friend Carlos Casagemas. Instantly I thought (as I believe the curator intended), "How profound." That pairing—melancholic/deep—is a central trope of the culture. Or to allude to another recent museum exhibition: for years the rap on Pierre Bonnard was that his paintings were too cheerful to be important. Here is the corresponding trope: happy/superficial.

Surely the central tenet of literary criticism is Franz Kafka's: "I think we ought to read only the kind of books that wound and stab us. . . . We need the books that affect us like a disaster, that grieve us deeply, like the death of someone we loved more than ourselves, like being banished into forests far from every one, like a suicide."[7] This need may even be pragmatic. In his poetry (I am thinking of "Terence, this is stupid stuff"), A. E. Housman argues that painful literature immunizes us against the pain of life's disappointments.

And here I want to lay down two linked challenges that are intentionally provocative. The first is to say that the literary aesthetic makes most sense in relation to a particular temperament (the melancholic, in which one feels great pain in response to loss) in a particular culture (one lacking technologies to prevent or diminish that pain). What if Mithradates had had an antidote, so that he did not require prophylactic arsenic and strychnine? Might poetry appropriate to the antidepressant era be more like beer drinking? And might that new art still prove authentic to the way of the world?

The second challenge is yet more provocative; call it intentionally hyperbolic: to say that there is no neutral venue for this debate over alienation or cosmesis because our sensibility has been largely formed by melancholics. Much of philosophy is written, and much art has been created, by melancholics or the outright depressed as a response to their substantial vulnerabilities. To put the matter only slightly less provocatively (and to return to the first challenge), much of philosophy is directed at depression as a threatening element of the human condition.

As Martha Nussbaum's *The Therapy of Desire* demonstrates in detail, classical moral philosophy is a means for coping with extremes of affect that follow upon loss.[8] The ancient Greeks' recommendations for the good life, in the writings of the Cynics and Stoics and Epicureans and Aristotelians, amount to ways to buffer the vicissitudes of attachment. If loss were less painful, the good life might be characterized not by *ataraxia* but by gusto. The connection between philosophy and melancholy continues in the medieval writings on *akadie* and then in the Enlightenment, through Montaigne and through Pascal, who writes, "Man is so unhappy that he would be bored even if he had no cause for boredom, by the very nature of his temperament."[9] In a study of Kierkegaard, Harvie Ferguson writes, "Modern philosophy, particularly in Descartes, Kant, and Hegel, presupposed as a permanent condition the melancholy of modern life."[10] Even those, like Kierkegaard, who chide melancholics do so from such a decided melancholic position that their writing reinforces the notion that melancholy is profundity. It is Kierkegaard who inspires Walker Percy, Kierkegaard whose body of work implies that melancholy is appropriate to modernity.

As for literature, studies indicate that an astonishing percentage, perhaps a vast majority, of serious writers are depressives. Researchers have speculated on the cause of that connection—Does depression put one in touch with important issues of deterioration and loss? But no one has asked what it means for us as a culture or even as a species that our unacknowledged legislators suffer from mood disorders, or something like. If there is no inherent moral distinction between melancholy and sanguinity, then we will need to worry about the association between creativity and mood. What if there is a consistent bias in the intellectual assessment of the good life or the wise perspective on life, an inherent bias against sanguinity hidden (and apparent) in philosophy and art?

An argument of this sort is worrisome—more worrisome than the conundrum we began with. Yet can we in good faith ignore the question of who sets the values? I have been, in effect, proposing still another thought experiment: Imagine a medication that diminishes the extremes of emotional response to loss, imparting the resilience already enjoyed by those with an even, sunny disposition. What would be the central philosophical questions in a culture where the use of this medication is widespread?

Aesthetic values do change in the light of changing views of health and illness. Elsewhere I have asked why we are no longer charmed by suicidal melancholics such as Goethe's Werther or Chateaubriand's René or Chekov's Ivanov.[11] Because we see major depression and affectively driven personality disorders as medically pathologic, what once exemplified authenticity now looks like immaturity or illness—as if the Romantic writers had made a category error.

A final thought experiment: Imagine that the association between melancholy and literary talent is based on a random commonality of cause: the genes for both cluster, say, side by side on a chromosome.

PETER D. KRAMER

Let us further imagine a culture in which melancholy, now clearly separate from creativity, is treated pharmacologically on a routine basis. In this culture, it is the melancholics manqués who write—melancholics rendered sanguine—so that the received notions of beauty and intimacy and nobility of character relate to bravado, decisiveness, and connections to social groups, not in the manner of false cheerleading but authentically, from the creative wellsprings of the optimistic.

What would be the notion of authenticity under such conditions? Perhaps in such a culture "strong evaluation" would find psychic resilience superior to alienation. Even today, many a melancholic looks at Panurge or Tom Jones with admiration—how marvelous to face the world with appetite! The notion of a sanguine culture horrifies those of us resonant with an aesthetics of melancholy, but morally, is such a culture inferior, assuming its art corresponds to the psychic reality? Is there a principled basis for linking melancholy to authenticity? Is there a moral hierarchy of temperaments?

I have offered an extreme version of an argument that might be more palatable in subtler form. I hope I have been convincing, or at least troubling, in one regard: the assertion that there is no privileged place to stand, no way to get outside the problem of authenticity as regards temperament.

Elliott asks whether we do not lose sight of something essential about ourselves when we see alienation and guilt as symptoms to be treated rather than as clues to our condition as human beings. The answer is in part empirical, in part contingent (on the social conditions of human life, a culture's technological resources, and such), and altogether aesthetic. If extremes of alienation are shown to arise from neuropathology, and if aspects of that pathology respond to treatment, our notion of the essential will change. And it may be that what remains of the experience and the concept of alienation will be yet more morally admirable—alienation stripped of compulsion, alienation independent of genetic happenstance, alienation that arises from free choice.

I want to end by saying that, like Percy and Elliott, in my private aesthetic I value depression and alienation, see them as postures that have salience for the culture and inherent beauty. But the role of philosophy is to question preferences. The case for and against alienation seems to me at this moment wide open. It has become easy, in the light of the debate over Prozac, to imagine material circumstances that might cause us to reassess which aspects of alienation fall into which category. The challenge of Prozac is precisely that it puts in question our tastes and values.

NOTES

1. Peter D. Kramer, *Listening to Prozac* (New York: Viking, 1993).

2. Carl Elliott, "The Tyranny of Happiness: Ethics and Cosmetic Psychopharmacology," in *Enhancing Human Traits: Ethical and Social Implications*, ed. Erik Parens (Washington, D.C.: Georgetown University Press, 1998), 183.

3. Walker Percy, *Lost in the Cosmos* (New York: Washington Square Press, 1983), 79, quoted in Carl Elliott, "Prozac and the Existential Novel: Two Therapies," in *The Last Physician: Walker Percy and the Moral Life of Medicine*, ed. Carl Elliott and John Lantos (Durham, N.C.: Duke University Press, 1999), 65.

4. Edmund Wilson, "Philocheles: The Wound and the Bow," in *The Wound and the Bow: Seven Studies in Literature* (Cambridge, Mass.: Riverside Press, 1941), 272–95; Lionel Trilling, *The Liberal Imagination: Essays on Literature and Society* (New York: Viking, 1950), 160–80.

5. Peter D. Kramer, introduction to *On Becoming a Person*, by Carl Rogers (Boston: Houghton Mifflin, 1995).

6. Elliott, "Tyranny of Happiness," 183.

7. Franz Kafka, letter to Oskar Pollak, January 27, 1904, in *Letters to Friends, Family, and Editors*, trans. Richard and Clara Winston (New York: Schocken Books, 1977), 16.

8. Martha C. Nussbaum, *The Therapy of Desire: Theory and Practice in Hellenistic Ethics* (Princeton: Princeton University Press, 1994).

9. Blaise Pascal, quoted in Harvie Ferguson, *Melancholy and the Critique of Modernity: Søren Kierkegaard's Religious Psychology* (London: Routledge, 1995), 25.

10. See ref. 7, Ferguson, *Melancholy and the Critique of Modernity*, 32.

11. Kramer, *Listening to Prozac*, 297, and Peter D. Kramer, "Stage View: What Ivanov Needs Is an Antidepressant," *New York Times*, December 21, 1997.

JAMES C. EDWARDS

Passion, Activity, and the Care of the Self
Foucault and Heidegger in the Precincts of Prozac

Mariah exploded with anger, her sentences flashing out into the shocked faces of her classmates. "I'm sick and tired of you guys, you *men*, telling me what I ought to think. It's *my* life, and if I want to make it better, that's my choice, not yours. Where does it say I have to put up with second-best? Where does it say *you* get to make the call?"

Airbursts of fury detonating in college classrooms are not unfamiliar occurrences, of course, and we can easily imagine a variety of provocations to call Mariah's words forth; but in order to understand this particular young woman's anger, you need to know that for three or four years now I have been teaching Peter Kramer's *Listening to Prozac* as one of the texts in my introductory philosophy course.[1] Pedagogically it is a good choice. Not only is the book engagingly written, full of both fascinating fact and compelling narrative, and not only is Kramer himself both philosophically and ethically astute, a voice well worth listening to, but the material he is recounting dovetails nicely with one of the course's central themes, which is what one might call *the ethic of authenticity*: the idea that one of the fundamental ethical tasks of every person is finding, nurturing, and elaborating a life that is distinctively her or his own, a life that exhibits, in Emerson's famous phrase, "self-reliance."[2]

It is easy to see how this theme—much on the minds of twenty-year-olds—gets played out in Kramer's book. Think of the transformation that occurs in the patient he calls "Tess." She, as you may remember, presented herself to Kramer as a clear case of depression, one he did not hesitate to treat with Prozac and psychotherapy. The course of that treatment was textbook smooth, just the sort of thing that the Eli Lilly folks (and their stockholders) had dreamed of. Tess was a classic "good responder." She went from being a harried, depressive, tired,

and lonely woman to being a fireball at work, a competent and solici-
tous parent, and a sexually attractive and confident lover—all because,
in her view, a little green-and-white capsule left a bit more serotonin
in her synapses for a bit longer.

An unmitigated success? Well, not according to lots of my students.
That is because Tess's case—apparently so well managed by her physician—had a sting in its tail. Once she had been free of her depression
for some months, Kramer, as is normal, gradually weaned her from
her medication, carefully checking to ensure the illness did not return.
It did not, thank goodness, but a few months later Tess reappeared at
his office to report that she was not satisfied with how she was feeling. She had lost her edge: her self-confidence was not what it had
been; things at work were not going so well; her thoughts seemed a
bit sluggish. In sum, she just did not like the way things were heading.
She put her distress to Kramer in a particularly poignant way: "I just
don't feel myself," she said. The Tess that she had been on Prozac now
seemed to her the *true* Tess, the one she always had it in herself to be.
Without the drug she was not ill (her definitively depressive symptoms had not returned, according to Kramer), but she also was not
satisfied. Prozac had, so to speak, reset her baseline of what counted
(to her) as her normal functioning. She wanted her physician to put
her back on the medication so that she could "be herself" again. (After
some hesitation, he did.)

Many (but not all) of my students find Tess's (and Kramer's) response distressing. They do not—I am glad to report—find it problematic to use Prozac to cure Tess's depression. They realize, some of
them from harsh firsthand experience, that depression is a serious and
frequently life-threatening illness, an illness just as physiological and
just as scary as cancer. If one is sick, one tries to get well using whatever therapies are safe and effective; that is a no-brainer. What bothers
them is that, as Kramer insists, Tess is not still sick. Her depression,
clinically defined, is gone; what she is feeling now is not symptom, it
is (her) reality. And she wants to change that reality with a drug. That
bothers lots of my students, and it bothers them even after it is pointed
out that Prozac is not one of those drugs that, so to speak, "masks"
reality to make it more palatable. It does not fool one about what is
real or take the sharp edges off things so they do not hurt anymore.
Quite the contrary: the drug seems only to make it possible for one
to face reality with energy, self-confidence, and focus. Tess's problems
do not disappear on Prozac, nor does she zone out and stop caring (for
a time) about her difficulties. On the medication she still has her life,

but now she is empowered to face it, to deal with it energetically and intelligently. But lots of my students are still not satisfied.

There are two quite different sources of their distress, what we can call, first, their *metaphysical worry* about Prozac and, second, their *ethical worry* about the drug. The metaphysical worry is that the remarkable effects of this medication confirm a commitment to what Kramer calls biological materialism, to the idea that we human beings are just interesting pieces of meat, nothing more and nothing less. When my students hear Tess saying, "I'm not myself" without the drug, and when they see from Kramer's cases how one's deepest sense of self-identity can be transformed by inhibited reuptake of serotonin, they find it hard to stick with their Cartesian distinction between mind and body; thus they also find it hard to hold onto such metaphysical convictions as the soul or free will, convictions they have lashed tightly (and usually uncritically) to their Cartesianism. Their view of the self begins to totter. Moreover, if Tess's identity is capable of being reconstructed by a drug, if (as she says) she is her "true self" only when taking Prozac, then what can we say about her—or anyone's—capacity for an authentic life, a life true to her own deepest individuality? For what would that "individuality" be? How can we make sense of the notion of a true self once we listen to the drug and its siren songs of effortless chemical change? Post-Prozac, how could "Who am I?" ever have a single, true answer? These questions cut deep into the metaphysics of the self, and Kramer's book nicely forces them upon us.

The ethical worry my students have about Tess's case is less easy to characterize. In the first instance it has to do with the fact, as they see it, that she is no longer *sick*. (As I have said, they do not doubt that depression is an illness and that illnesses need to be cured—with drugs, with surgery, or with whatever is appropriate.) So if Tess is not sick, then what is going on? It must be that she just wants to be *different*, to be *happier*. This case (they think) is not any longer about cure; it is about self-transformation. At that point their ethical worry takes the form of two prejudices they are quick to voice (and slow to defend): when it comes to changing one's life (1) the natural way is better than the artificial, and (2) the hard way is better than the easy. (I call these prejudices just to mark the immediate and largely thoughtless way they are presented in discussion; I am not assuming that, suitably formulated, they contain no truth whatsoever.) My students claim to have no objections to Tess's self-transformation if it were done through some sort of "talking cure," whether psychological, philosophical, or religious. They would be glad for her to diet strenuously; to undertake a rigorous program of exercise, meditation, and prayer; to see a therapist once a week; or to read Plato, the Bible, and Deepak Chopra. All these things are (to them) "natural" avenues of self-transformation.[3] And—this is important, I believe—whatever gain these methods purchase requires its corresponding pain. Good puritans that my students are, they know that life is deep and serious and costly; nothing good comes to one without its required agony. (Even if they are not Christians, the cross is never far from their minds. I live and teach in the South, remember.) So Tess is for these folks a figure of weakness, of shortcut. Either she should hunker down to some serious (i.e., painful and natural) work of therapy or she should accept her limitations and get on with her life as it is.

Thus Mariah's outburst: she saw these objections, made mostly and most vociferously in my classes by men, as counsels of despair motivated by the desire to, if not actually to keep women "in their place" of self-distrust, melancholy, and fatigue, then at least to insist that their way out of the valley of the shadow be appropriately heroic and "masculine." ("Go the bloody *hard* way," Ludwig Wittgenstein was fond of adjuring his students.) Mariah was having none of this. For her, Tess was an exemplary figure: a woman who had with Kramer's help asserted control over her life and who now wanted to extend that control on her own, with the help of Prozac. For Mariah, and for her reading of Tess, Prozac is a drug of liberation, and maybe especially of women's liberation.

I suspect there is nothing particularly surprising to us about Mariah's reaction, and I recount it here only to remind myself (and perhaps you, if you need it) that first-order moralizing about "enhancement technologies" such as Prozac is a tricky and sometimes dangerous business. In this sort of case it is unlikely that our thinking turns on simple choices between stark principles, on the sorts of binary, one-zero decisions that ethical theorists are taught—or used to be taught—to revere. What we think about Tess's continued use (and Kramer's continued prescription) of Prozac past the cure of her illness will not, for me, happily resolve itself either into a principled preference for natural forms of self-transformation or into a principled conviction that access to personal empowerment is always a good thing for a woman. No, my own intuitions here have less to do with definitively moral principles and choices and more to do with larger-scale concepts and their strains of commitment, concepts that are at best quasi-ethical. In particular, what makes a case like Tess's so interesting and so dif-

JAMES C. EDWARDS

ficult is—I find—how my reactions to Tess and to Kramer are bound up with the large concepts of activity and passion. Those concepts are bound up in their turn, sometimes in quite messy ways, with ideas about disease and health, about masculinity and femininity, and ultimately about good and evil themselves. In the course of this single essay I cannot hope to sort out all the messes, but together we might at least make a start.

Consider these sentences from Michel Foucault's third volume of his *History of Sexuality, The Care of the Self*:

> In keeping with a tradition that goes back a very long way in Greek culture, the care of the self is in close correlation with medical thought and practice. This ancient correlation became increasingly strong, so much so that Plutarch is able to say, at the beginning of *Advice about Keeping Well*, that philosophy and medicine are concerned with a "single field" *(mia chora)*. They do draw on a shared set of notions, whose central element is the concept of pathos. It applies to passion as well as to physical illness, to the distress of the body and to the involuntary movement of the soul; and in both cases alike, it refers to a state of passivity, which for the body takes the form of a disorder which upsets the balance of its humors or its qualities and which for the soul takes the form of a movement capable of carrying it away in spite of itself. On the basis of this shared concept, it was possible to construct a grid of analysis that was valid for the ailments of the body and the soul.[4]

Notice how, in Foucault's account, ideas about passion and activity are deeply implicated in conceptions of disease and health, both physical and spiritual. The care of the self, which is the defining ambition of philosophy, and the care of the body, which is the defining ambition of medicine, are both characterized as the conquest—however temporary—of "pathos." The philosopher and the physician equally struggle against an "involuntary movement," a disorder that presses itself upon one from "outside" (so to speak), upsetting the internally regulated and harmonious balance of forces that is, in the ideal, one's natural activity. Health, whether of the body or of the soul, is pictured here as a certain sort of imperviousness, a capacity to resist depredations upon one's internal ordering of oneself. To be well is to exercise a particular sort of self-generated and well-ordered self-determination. To be easily moved, and especially to be subject to involuntary movement, is dangerous; to submit to pathos is to open oneself to disturbance and disease.

It is tempting to dismiss Foucault's claims by saying they are interesting as historical analysis but useless as contemporary heuristic. "Maybe"—so speaks the protesting voice—"that was the way some of the Stoics thought about disease and health; but *we moderns*, possessed of much more detailed and accurate physiological accounts of disease-etiology, *we* don't think about wellness as orderly internal self-determination, nor do we identify 'pathos' as the master concept of illness." But the protest here is hollow, since of course we often *do* think this way, at least at the level of linguistic trope. (And what level is deeper than that, after all?) In what we typically say, in the ordinary forms of our talk with one another, we constantly find ourselves conceiving of illness as something that besets us against our will, as a disequilibrating force from outside our natural ordering, an external force against which we struggle to free ourselves. "Don't get too close; I'm fighting a cold," we caution our neighbor. Or we report, "John's depression really has him by the throat these days." Or as children we tell a silly joke to explain why we got sick: "I slept with the window open and in-flew-enza." All these banal locutions (and their banality is here just the point) picture the illness as an external force, a disorder that sets upon us—and thereby moves us involuntarily off our normal and orderly path. Likewise, we counsel ourselves and others not to give in to the disease we are struggling with, to repel the viral or cellular invasion aggressively, to marshal our T-cells to our defense. We suffer our illnesses, as we say, and that does not (just) mean that they often cause us pain. It means that we *bear* them; they come to us as passions to be undergone,[5] as burdens laid on us, willy-nilly, from outside our natural course of orderly and self-determined activity. Even our words "pathology" and "pathogen" enshrine the ancient idea that pathos is essentially linked to disease. All these familiar grammatical pictures play into just the dynamic of passion/activity that Foucault identifies as central to ancient medicine and philosophy.[6] In this way we are closer to Plutarch than we might want to think.

How would Foucault's analysis of the depth grammar of disease and health construe Tess's story? Well, when Tess was ill with her depression, she was in the grip of a passion, an involuntary movement of the body and soul; that is, she was moved off her normal (self-regulating, self-determining) course through life by the onset of a force from outside that normal course, a force that slowed her down, that sapped her energy and hope, that deflected her from her ordinary aims, and that diminished her capacity for self-possession. Happily, under treatment with Prozac and psychotherapy, this disordering force was conquered, or at least repelled. Tess was no longer suffering, no longer subject to involuntary movement, to pathos. She was again in orderly possession of herself; she was well.

What about later, when she returned to Kramer saying that she "wasn't herself" and wanting him to prescribe more of the drug? Here the grammar of passion and pathos does not have nearly so much traction as before. At this point it is harder for us to see that Tess is in the grip of an involuntary movement that is deflecting her from her normal course of self-regulating, self-determining behavior. After all, we can see, as Kramer did, that she is doing pretty well with her life; she is not just about to go under. Maybe she is not playing at the top of her game anymore, but that does not indicate true *pathology*, does it? (How many of us play consistently at the top level, after all; and are we *ill*?) Whatever Tess does at this point does not seem to be about illness and health. Thus we begin to talk about enhancement rather than cure, and with that change particular ethical problems for the first time begin to arise. Here my students begin to voice their anxious objections to the use of a drug to tweak personality—to be the "chemical crutch" Tess leans on, and so forth.

But also here the categories of passion and activity come up in another way to shape our ethical thinking. For why should my students object to Tess's chemically produced enhancement? One possible source of such objection, and this (I believe) is what Mariah sensed in my class, is connected to some all-too-common prejudices about gender. For do we not, some of us, distrust and fear the attempts of women to enhance themselves, especially when such enhancement is at the woman's own control and when it seems to require no suffering or difficulty to be undergone? I suspect that some of our ambivalence about a drug like Prozac arises from the way it helps a person, especially a woman, to break free of passion, of involuntary movement, of suffering, of undergoing, and to become more active, more in control. Maybe it is not the happiness or the brightness we distrust as Prozac's products; maybe what we really distrust is the way those things seem to be cut free from pathos, the way they do not seem to have been earned by suffering.

Maybe that distrust is even stronger when the person in question is a woman, since—and I report this only as the vicious prejudice I believe it to be—women are supposed to be, or naturally are, more passionate than men. Women, after all, are supposed to suffer, in every sense of that rich term: they feel more; they bear more; they are more moved than we men are. It is one thing—this is what Mariah heard, or thought she heard, in my class—for a man to take control of himself, to order himself in orderly ways for the ordering of things. After all, that is what men do: they construct and run the world, and that requires moving things around in an orderly way, not being moved by them. Men have to be tough, impervious, capable of passing through the storms unscathed. That is the price they pay for ruling. But women, on the other hand, are creatures of passion, of heightened sensibility; they register things rather than rule them. They are beings of affection: they are affected by what is there, moved by it, and they somehow spread that affection around as loving-kindness. After class one day I was walking back to my office with an intro student who said, "Tess just wanted too much to succeed in her job. That's what got her back to Kramer wanting more Prozac. A job shouldn't be that important to someone." (I do not need to tell you that my student was a man, do I?) And you already know what I said in return, don't you?: "Would you feel the same way if it were Kramer's patient Sam, the architect, making the same plea?" I am glad to say my student had heart enough to be embarrassed by the question.

Although I am convinced that Mariah is correct and that some of our ambivalence about the use of Prozac as an enhancement technology has to do with gender prejudices about passion and activity that still haunt us, it would be too simple to leave the matter there. It is not just our (male) fear of *women* free of pathos that is in play here (though surely that is some of it); it is that none of us, women or men, really know the proper place of pathos in life. We are not a culture that is at peace with suffering things. By that I do not just mean that none of us likes to hurt; that, after all, seems both rational and good. I mean that we do not have a settled view about what virtue there is, or might be, in simply bearing things, in living in such a way that our ambition, or at least one of our ambitions, is to be open to things and events in such a way that we become their bearers; we become the places they appear and unfold. Rather than seeing ourselves as fundamentally (or only) agents, those who in an orderly way order things for the sake of (their/our) order, we could see ourselves more as persons who, through practices of deliberate acknowledgment, make it possible for things to register themselves, for events and entities to be present in all their richness.

The philosopher who has thought most deeply about this currently unfamiliar possibility, which he calls *Gelassenheit* ("letting-be"), is Martin Heidegger, and it is certainly not possible here to give a large-scale account of his work, or even of that (later) part of it that deals most directly with these matters.[7] Suffice it to say that for Heidegger the way of life called *Gelassenheit* is to be contrasted with a way of life that valorizes *die Technik*, "technology," and the life of technology is the kind of life that since at least the seventeenth century and the rise of its New Sciences we in the West have been living.

For most of us the word "technology" calls to mind the use of machines and tools, especially machines and tools powered by non-human sources of energy, to attain and to further human interests. But for Heidegger that is too simple an account: the key is to see *die Technik* as a way of revealing things, a way of letting something come to presence. Technology brings things into presence—lets them be seen—in a particular way; it reveals them as having a particular character, a particular Being.

The characteristic kind of thing brought to light by the practices of technology is *Bestand*, "standing-reserve": that which in an orderly way awaits our use of it for the further ordering of things. When I walk to my study in the morning and glance at the computer on the desk, the computer, as the thing it is, is *Bestand*. It reveals itself to me as waiting patiently for me to turn it on, to "get its things in order," so I can use it to order and reorder those things and others. The data stored there—words, sentences, thoughts, and bank balances—await my command so they can be transformed, distributed, and switched about: they, too, are *Bestand*. And it is not just the glass-and-plastic machines that reveal themselves to me as standing-reserve. As I glance out the window onto the leaves I have not yet raked, they, too, are *Bestand*: they patiently await my collection of them so they can be put onto the compost heap (stored up so the energy in them can later be unlocked) or bagged for the garbage collection (switched about). The very house I inhabit is, as we have famously been told, "a machine for living in," with the window out of which I gaze a device for the orderly collection of light (and the orderly retention of heat). The house patiently awaits its tenants for their use of it in ordering their lives; the land on which the house sits reveals itself through the window as garden and as landscape, waiting for the orderly touch that shapes and preserves and cultivates. The mugs on the kitchen shelf, the television in the loft, the cereal in the pantry, the toothbrush on the bathroom sink: all stand by in the manner of stock, as resources awaiting their call to orderly use in the ordering of things.

For us (almost) everything reveals itself as *Bestand*. Most of the time, of course, we are not explicitly aware that our things have that sort of Being. Our consciousness of them as standing-reserve shows itself not in anything we explicitly say or think about them; rather, it shows itself in how we comport ourselves to them in unselfconscious everyday action and reaction. How I see my television set or my coffee mug or my toothbrush shows itself in the way I carelessly handle these things, in the way my eye passes over them without a pause, in the way I irritably react when they do not perform as expected, in the thoughtless way I dispose of them when they are no longer useful, and so forth.

The appearance of things as *Bestand* is the inevitable result of those social practices that have as their nature and point what Heidegger calls ordering. What is this ordering? The dominant social practices constituting our world are practices that enframe: they are practices that put things in their proper places in such a way that they are readily available to be put to use by us with a maximum of efficiency and a minimum of attention to the conditions of their appearing. Such practices impose a grid (*Gestell*, "frame") upon things so that within that grid—within the completely and immediately surveyable space created by that grid—those things are completely and immediately locatable and thus are completely and immediately available for whatever use we find it appropriate to put them to. In this way things are made orderly. They are located within a frame that transparently orients us to them and them to us; as a result of that perspicuous orientation within the frame they are ours to use and reuse easily and quickly and essentially thoughtlessly. And the point of our use of our orderly things is further ordering. Under the spell of technology, we come to order things primarily for the sake of ordering itself.

It is hard not to recognize one's life in this (all-too-brief) Heideggerian sketch. It is also hard not to see enhancement technologies, in all their variety, as almost entirely defined by their contribution to the self required by this life of ordering. But I do not want to moralize this matter in any crude way: there is nothing obviously wrong with wanting a life of orderly activity that aims at the ordering of things so that they better serve our interests in various kinds of order. There's nothing obviously wrong with wanting to enframe the world, conceptually and otherwise. This, after all, is the life most of us lead and want. What is the alternative, after all? What would a life not essentially technological look like?

I do not have a full-fledged answer to that question, much less the time to deploy it if I did, but it is clear that it would be a life of pathos. A life of *Gelassenheit*, of letting things be, would be a life devoted not to orderly control *of* one's reactions so as to preserve one's capacity for orderly self-determination; it would be a life that welcomes and registers the disorder that comes when one fully registers the impacts *of* things upon one. It would be a life that conceives of itself less as the creation of something hard and enduring not already there and more as the increasingly plastic and receptive medium in which things leave their marks and traces. It would be a life that aims most centrally not at control and order but at "truth," at *alethia*, at passionately showing forth ("dis-closing") the conditions of the life one is actually living. In Heidegger's view such a life would be passionate but not passive, since the happening of truth always requires the making of things that bear that truth. *Gelassenheit* does not require hunkering down and giving up; it is not an invitation to death. But it does require a kind of surrender of oneself, a surrender of oneself into a kind of activity that aims not at ordering but at full acknowledgment. The poet, says Heidegger, is not the one who wills but the one who is willing—willing to release oneself into the draft of things and to be their witness.[8]

At another place I have tried to suggest some examples of such a life, a life in which the imagination—conceived of now as that still pool in which various figures show themselves to us and to themselves— is central.[9] I will not try to cover this ground again now, but for me the most compelling figure of such a life is Henry David Thoreau, or (better put) the author of *Walden*. The crucial thing to see in such an example is that the life of *Gelassenheit* is not a life of passivity or inactivity. On the contrary, Thoreau builds a house and hoes beans and writes poems and measures the depth of the pond and . . . . But the point of these activities is not, sad to say, the point of what I typically do in my life. Thoreau is not, I think, trying to create order, to hold chaos at bay, to make himself victorious over his shortcomings and the shortcomings of the world as he finds it. His point is not enhancement—not enhancement of anything. His point is to be a truthful witness, a place where the gods appear, and for that, pathos is required. For that, one must cultivate the imagination, the pool whose waters may be roiled by the presence of the unseen. A person whose aim is that sort of receptivity, who courts that sort of disturbance and disorder, holy and unholy, will not be a person who cares much about training for the sort of race that most of us are running.

Again I want to make it clear that one cannot despise the life of *die Technik*, unless one is willing to despise oneself, and such self-hatred, or (more likely) pretense of self-hatred, is not attractive. We cannot look at Tess and say, "She ought not want to succeed. She ought not want to play at the top of her game. In fact, she ought not want to play that game at all." In the same way, we cannot look someone in the face and say, "You ought not want straighter teeth or clearer skin or more hair or less abdominal fat or better vision or a quicker mind or a better memory or . . . ." How can we, who have (some) of these advantages—advantages in the games we indeed play—moralize carelessly about the others who want them? When that moralizing starts to happen, one looks around—as Mariah astutely did—for some reasons for it, reasons having to do with cui bono; usually they are not far to seek. I am just as vulnerable to such self-serving moralizing as anyone else, but here I want to try to resist it.

The point for us is not to insist on one of these lives in preference to the other; still less is it for us to evangelize—for others—that life that none of us actually leads. The point is, first, to realize that there are at least two sorts of lives there to be lived, to realize that our common sense, and common life, is a historical construction, not the plain sense of things. This, I think, is Heidegger's virtue: he reminds us—he said his sort of thinking was *Andenken* ("recollection," "memorializing")—that the life of technological ordering is not the only life there has been. Even if we are not yet in position to take its measure, and to measure it against the life we ordinarily live (and I think we are *not* ready to do that), such measuring will come only when the alternatives are clear to us. Thus the philosophical work we need to do is not, as we might think, to find within our ordinary ethical lives the wherewithal to say yea or nay about Prozac or other enhancement technologies, and it is not even to deprecate those lives in favor of some other, radically altered version of them. Both those reactions, the complacent and the eschatological, strike me as too easy, and too easily seductive. (We all know the seductive power, on one hand, of good common sense ["rigorous, analytical thinking"] and, on the other, of turning over the fruit basket ["Only a god can save us!"].)[10] I think we need to do something slower, more difficult, and probably less attractive. (Certainly it will be harder to get on television, or to do consultations, with this as one's commitment.) What we need to be doing is to explore, sensibly and carefully and critically, the possibility that we—some of us—can and should live differently than we do. Until we have done that, and until we ourselves have experimented with what we have discovered, I suspect we will stay pretty much on the surface of the problems we would like to resolve.

As long as (almost) all we could expect medicine to do was cure illness, then we did not have to wrestle with our ambivalence about pathos. To get rid of pain and disability does not, ceteris paribus, cause

JAMES C. EDWARDS

us ethical qualm. But now we can do more, and we are expected to. Now medicine has become a full part of the *die Technik*, in a way that goes far beyond just the use of powerful and complicated machines to make diagnosis and cure easier. Now medicine—Prozac, liposuction, Propecia—is one more arrow in the quiver of those of us who go out every day to bring back meat to the table or, to use Richard Wilber's less violent, more agricultural metaphor, to milk the cow of the world. Perhaps we should be glad of that—bemoaning it does no good anyway—since maybe our immersion in technology and its discontents will provoke a more careful examination of what alternatives to it there still may be.

NOTES

1. Peter D. Kramer, *Listening to Prozac* (New York: Penguin, 1994).

2. Ralph Waldo Emerson, "Self-reliance," in the Library of America volume devoted to Emerson, pp. 259–82. In this connection, see also Charles Taylor, *The Ethics of Authenticity* (Cambridge, Mass.: Harvard University Press).

3. It is a fascinating question, of course, why they see some methods of self-transformation as natural and others as artificial. Part of the answer certainly has simply to do with what they are used to, but I do not think that is all that is involved. I will not chase this rabbit in this essay.

4. Michel Foucault, *The Care of the Self*, trans. Robert Hurley (New York: Vintage, 1988), 54.

5. Think, in this connection, of the Passion of Jesus, the pain and death he had to undergo, to suffer: passion is "pathos."

6. For an account of grammatical pictures and the role they play in philosophical perplexity, see Ludwig Wittgenstein, *Philosophical Investigations*, trans. G. E. M. Anscombe (Oxford: Basil Blackwell, 1953). I have tried to extend Wittgenstein's remarks in *Ethics without Philosophy: Wittgenstein and the Moral Life* (Gainesville: University Presses of Florida, 1982).

7. For a discussion of these matters, see my *The Plain Sense of Things: The Fate of Religion in an Age of Normal Nihilism* (University Park, Pa.: Penn State Press, 1997).

8. Martin Heidegger, "What Are Poets For?," in *Poetry, Language, Truth*, trans. Albert Hofstadter (New York: Harper and Row, 1971).

9. See Edwards, *Plain Sense of Things*, chap. 5, for details.

10. The phrase is from Heidegger's notorious interview with *Der Spiegel*, published posthumously in 1976, showing that even he on occasion succumbed to the siren song of eschatology.

DAVID HEALY

Good Science or Good Business?

When *Listening to Prozac* emerged in 1993, it was one of the few books dealing with psychiatry to become an international best seller since Freud's and Jung's works, and the only book on psychopharmacology ever to do so. The book dealt with the effects of an "antidepressant" on conditions that often looked more like states of alienation than classic depressions. For many, this was their first awareness that antidepressants were drugs distinguishable from minor tranquilizers. For others, Peter Kramer's book and the notion of cosmetic psychopharmacology that it introduced raised interesting ethical and philosophical dilemmas. But the argument here is that the attraction of the book has depended on a series of engineered transformations in the way we think about mental well-being. The "alienation" Prozac and similar therapies "treat" has very commonly been defined in terms of the interests of the medico-pharmaceutical complex, and the arguments offered about the merits of Prozac look more like descriptions of the interests of their proponents than dependable accounts of reality.

The interface between mental health and alienation traces to the emergence of psychodynamic therapy at the turn of the twentieth century, but this new industry remained at one remove from psychiatry until the 1950s. While the therapists took charge of such problems as alienation, psychiatrists dealt with those suffering from fullblown psychoses. In the interim, there was considerable recourse to do-it-yourself pharmaco-"therapy" that employed alcohol, opiates, bromides, and barbiturates to manage community nervousness (that is, nervous conditions that do not lead to hospitalization). But this use, unconstrained by a therapy establishment, gave rise to little talk of alienation among the philosophers. Indeed one can wonder whether many philosophy departments would be able to function without alcohol to facilitate social intercourse.

When imipramine, the first antidepressant, was introduced, clinicians and pharmaceutical company executives could see little rationale for it. The frequency of affective disorders appeared vanishingly low, and these conditions responded to antipsychotics or electroconvulsive therapy. Clinicians used the antidepressants sparingly, and the very word "antidepressant" began to appear in dictionaries only in the mid-1980s.[1] Unlike the antipsychotics, the antidepressants had no clear niche. However, they did seem capable of making some difference to a large number of people, even if those people might have to be persuaded that they needed this difference in their lives. As early as 1958, Roland Kuhn, the discoverer of imipramine, had noted that some sexual perversions responded to imipramine and that many patients, when they recovered, felt better than well.[2] Such transformations opened up significant philosophical and ethical issues—claims now strongly suggestive of Kramer's agenda. But whereas Kramer's book became a runaway best seller, Kuhn's speculations had minimal impact. The philosophers who were excited by the new psychotropic compounds in the 1950s and are now interested in neuroscience and Prozac were not interested in imipramine.

MARKET DEVELOPMENT

The developmental trajectory for the antidepressants was largely determined by a critical external event: the thalidomide disaster. The public reaction to the birth defects caused by thalidomide, which had been taken by pregnant women to combat "morning sickness," led to the 1962 Food and Drug Act amendments, which channeled drug development toward clear diseases. Drug availability was restricted to prescription-only medicines, placing it in the hands of individuals who supposedly would make drugs available for problems stemming only from diseases rather than for those stemming from other sources. These developments radically changed psychiatry, first, by putting a premium on "categorical" rather than "dimensional" models of disease, so that psychiatrists were more likely to treat diseases as conditions that patients either have or lack rather than have to some degree, and second, because prescription-only status brought nervousness within the psychiatric ambit.

Initially, the straitjacket of the 1962 amendments had the outcomes intended. But if drugs are made available only for diseases, it was perhaps predictable that there would be a mass creation of disease. There has been, and these developments shape our perceptions of how alienation is being managed. In the 1950s, it was thought that only 50 people per million were depressed. Nowadays no one blinks on being told that depression affects more than 100,000 per million and that it leads to more disability and economic disadvantage than any other disorder.[3] But this change plainly requires a major change in our view of what constitutes disease. If 10 to 15 percent of the population is depressed, the label "disease" does not make sense if understood in terms of the biological disruption that bacterial infections produce. What is meant can be grasped only if the "disease state" is framed in terms of temperamental factors and only if what is aimed at is a state of comparative well-being rather than cure.

Oddly enough, the widespread acceptance of our views of depression conceals the process by which they were changed. When first faced with the question of what community nervousness is, the psychiatric profession and the pharmaceutical industry understood it in terms of anxiety, and they resorted to Valium and other anxiolytics to treat it. This led to the first debates about the ethics of treating "problems of living" in this way.[4] In the West, however, the 1980s crisis surrounding benzodiazepine dependence led to the eclipse of both the minor tranquilizers and the whole notion of anxiolysis. This ushered in the antidepressant era. In contrast, in Japan, where dependence is less of a problem, the anxiolytics remain the most widely used drugs for nervousness and the antidepressant market remains small. Depression as it is now understood by clinicians and at street level is therefore an extremely recent phenomenon, largely confined to the West. Its emergence coincides with the development of the selective serotonin reuptake inhibitors (SSRIs), which in the mid-1980s appeared capable of development as either anxiolytics or antidepressants.[5] Since their initial launch as antidepressants, various SSRIs have been approved for the treatment of panic disorder, social phobia, posttraumatic stress disorder, obsessive-compulsive disorder, and other anxiety-based conditions. In a number of these disorders, the SSRIs are more effective than they are in depression. Indeed, it has not been possible to show that Prozac is effective in classic depressive disorders. Worse, there is some evidence that far from reducing rates of suicide and disability associated with depression, antidepressants may actually increase them. Prozac and related drugs are prescribed to more than 4 million children and teenagers per annum in the United States, yet a preponderance of evidence suggests that such prescriptions are not warranted.[6]

The designation of Prozac as an antidepressant means that some efficacy in some milder depressions can be shown for this compound, and it is accordingly not illegal to market it as a treatment for depression; but the fact that Prozac "works" for some people does not mean

DAVID HEALY

that they have classic depression. That it was marketed this way stems from business rather than scientific calculations.[7] Changes in the way we think about problems of living are not restricted to depression. The research demonstrating that SSRIs could be useful for treating other nervous conditions has been associated with marked increases in estimates of their frequency as well.[8] Obsessive-compulsive disorder has increased a thousandfold in apparent frequency. "Panic disorder," a term coined in the mid-1960s and first appearing in diagnostic classification systems in 1980, has become one of the most widely recognized psychiatric terms at street level. Social phobia, all but invisible until the 1990s, now appears to affect the population in such epidemic proportions that the launch of Paxil as an antishyness agent was a media event.

These changes have very likely been brought about by the pharmaceutical industry itself, through its highly developed capacities for gathering and disseminating evidence germane to its business interests. The methods that might have this effect include convening consensus conferences and publishing the proceedings, sponsoring symposia at professional meetings, and funding special supplements to professional journals. The industry may also establish and support patient groups to lobby for treatments. The claim here—though defended elsewhere—is that these and other techniques for marketing information are sufficiently well developed that significant changes in the mentality of both clinicians and the public can be produced within a few years.[9] In effect, the industry has educated prescribers and the public to recognize many other kinds of cases as depression.

These changes are facilitated by a broader social shift. When dynamic therapies occupied the citadels of orthodoxy in psychiatry, their terminology leaked out into popular language. A variety of terms were used in ways that technically were wholly inaccurate but that nevertheless became part of how we thought of ourselves and conceptualized alienation. Recently, the psychobabble prevalent during much of the twentieth century has begun to give ground to a newly minted biobabble. A rootless patois of biological terms—"low brain amines," for example—has settled into the popular consciousness, with consequences for our self-conception that can only be guessed at.[10]

Possibly, Prozac's success has also depended partly on a lack of information. Prozac has been shown to "work" using clinician-based, disease-specific rating scales, but when patient-based, nonspecific quality of life instruments have been used, it has not been shown to work for depression—although this information has not seen the light of day.[11] Current methods to estimate the side effects of drugs in clinical trials actually underestimate them, according to some tallies, by a sixfold factor.[12] Finally, the SSRIs have been sold on the back of a claim that the claim of suicide is 600 per every 100,000 patient years. But this is the rate for people with severe depression, for which Prozac does not work. The rate for primary care depression is on the order of 30 out of every 100,000 people. Yet in these populations, suicide rates of 189 for every 100,000 on Prozac have been reported.[13] Thus there are good grounds to believe that Prozac can trigger suicidality. The pharmaceutical companies are not investigating, however; one wonders whether they are receiving legal advice echoing that given to the tobacco companies, that any investigation of these issues may increase product liability. From this vantage point, Prozac might seem better cast as a symbol of the alienation that large corporations can visit on people rather than as a symbol of the "treatment" of alienation that a psychotropic agent can bring about.

LIFESTYLES AND THE DISEASE MODEL

The public perception of Prozac, as shaped by *Listening to Prozac*, was that the drug had been rationally engineered, in the sense that it had been developed so as to achieve highly reproducible clinical outcomes. If it is important that a drug be rationally engineered, it seems clear that Kuhn's discovery of cosmesis, in contrast to Kramer's, could not have gone anywhere.

However, Kramer's mythic account of the development of Prozac was mistaken. It was perhaps prophetic, since neuroimaging technologies, pharmacogenetic techniques, and other novel strategies will make the development of psychotropic drugs increasingly rational in this industrial sense, but none of this applied to Prozac. While Prozac works for some people, it has not been possible to offer any guarantees as to the quality of clinical outcomes when using it. Lacking such guarantees does not matter as much in treating genuine disease, since when patients are in danger, even doing something risky is by consensus preferable to doing nothing. But poor outcomes are much less tolerable in the management of less severe conditions. Thus a disease model offers pharmaceutical companies and clinicians a valuable escape from quality standards.

A disease model offers other advantages to pharmaceutical companies. It acts powerfully to legitimate drug-taking, allowing Prozac, for example, to escape the flak that Valium drew in the 1970s. And it can function as a means of resolving problems about equitable access to health resources, since it is widely accepted that there are greater difficulties with inequities in health care than with inequities in the access to computers or digital televisions.

Prozac is of course only one of a growing number of agents that modulate lifestyles rather than cure diseases. Viagra is another good example of this trend. Viagra's designation as a lifestyle agent depends in good part on the reliability with which the intended responses can be elicited. What is interesting about Viagra is that we have had other drugs for at least two decades that have comparable effects on sexual function. The SSRIS may have weak and unpredictable effects on depression, but they can reliably delay orgasm, and other antidepressants can advance it.[14] Thus we have had the capacity to "engineer" sexual performance for some time; the pharmaceutical companies have simply not marketed pills for such uses, presumably because they were uncertain about the acceptability of a "lifestyle market" for their wares.[15] Seen against this background, the promotion of Viagra marks an important turning point in the way drugs are developed.

In general, clinical therapeutics is increasingly comprised of a series of domains removed to varying degrees from the management of bacterial infections. The provision of oral contraceptives on a prescription-only basis is notionally underpinned by a disease model. Hormone replacement therapy is likewise presented as treatment for a disease. "Treatments" for baldness, age-induced skin changes, obesity, and a range of other lifestyle agents wait in the wings. All of these raise the question of what qualifies as a disease. In recent history, a disease has been thought of as an entity established by an underlying biological lesion. Previously, illnesses were anything that made the individual feel less well, a definition that potentially included halitosis. Latterly, the emergence of agents that can modify natural variations in hair loss or ejaculatory latency push us closer to making explicit one of the currently implicit but increasingly important definitions of disease, which is that it is, in practice, something that third-party payers will reimburse on.

Before 1962, tonics flourished along with treatments for halitosis and other problems of living. Cyproheptadine, an imipramine-like agent, which reliably improves appetite and sleep and less reliably cures depressions, was on sale as a tonic. The 1962 amendments required redesignation of agents like this as antidepressants rather than tonics, but in many ways, they might have had greater public acceptability if classified as tonics, a usage hallowed by centuries of practice, rather than as antidepressants, since as drugs they quickly became associated with risks of addiction. Would we be talking about alienation if it were over-the-counter tonics rather than prescription-only antidepressants that were involved—or if we were, would the public take our debate seriously? Could it be that much of the current debate is predicated on a combination of pseudoscientific mystique and regulatory artifact? Consider in this connection one of the dilemmas raised by Kramer: because of its prescription-only status, Prozac raises special moral problems for the physician, who is now called upon to decide whether it would be a good thing to reduce the general level of melancholy in the community, with the consequent loss of spirituality or creativity that might go with that.

These dilemmas would be transformed if the power to make these decisions were returned to the consumer. We may be unwittingly alienated choosing to purchase automobiles, but we would certainly feel alienated if it were the prerogative of the automobile salesmen to decide which brand of vehicle we should get.

NOTES

Editors' Note: Controversy has surrounded Healy's position on Prozac. Following the publication of his views in the *Hastings Center Report*, the pharmaceutical firm Eli Lilly withdrew its financial support of the Hastings Center. The University of Toronto also withdrew an offer of a faculty position after learning of his viewpoint on this issue. To read Healy's perspective on these events, see David Healy, "Conflicting Interests in Toronto," *Perspectives in Biology and Medicine* 45 (2002): 250–63.

1. D. Healy, "The Three Faces of the Antidepressants," *Journal of Nervous and Mental Disease* 187 (1999): 174–80.

2. R. Kuhn, "The Treatment of Depressive States with G22355 (Imipramine Hydrochloride)," *American Journal of Psychiatry* 115 (1958): 459–64.

3. C. Murray and A. Lopez, *The Global Burden of Disease* (Cambridge, Mass.: Harvard University Press, 1996).

4. M. C. Smith, *A Social History of the Minor Tranquillizers* (Binghamton, N.Y.: Haworth Press, 1991).

5. D. Healy and D. Nutt, "Prescriptions, Licences and Evidence," *Psychiatric Bulletin* 22 (1998): 680–84; D. Healy, "The Marketing of 5HT," *British Journal of Psychiatry* 158 (1991): 737–42.

6. Healy, "Marketing of 5HT."

7. R. L. Fisher and S. Fisher, "Antidepressants for Children: Is Scientific

Support Necessary? (With commentary by L. Eisenberg and E. Pellegrino)," *Journal of Nervous and Mental Disease* 184 (1996): 98–108.

8. D. Healy, *The Antidepressant Era* (Cambridge, Mass.: Harvard University Press, 1997).

9. For a full defense, see ibid.

10. E. S. Valenstein, *Blaming the Brain* (New York: Free Press, 1998).

11. Healy, "Three Faces of the Antidepressants."

12. S. Stecklow and L. Johannes, "Questions Arise on New Drug Testing: Drug Makers Relied on Clinical Researchers Who Now Await Trial," *Wall Street Journal*, August 15, 1997.

13. D. Healy et al., "Suicide in the Course of the Treatment of Depression," *Journal of Psychopharmacology* 13 (1999): 94–99.

14. Healy, *Antidepressant Era*.

15. Ibid.

FINANCIAL DISCLOSURE

In recent years David Healy has had consultancies with, been a principal investigator or trialist for, been a chairman or speaker at international symposia for, or received support to attend meetings from AstraZenca, Boots/ Knoll Pharmaceuticals, Eli Lilly, Janssen-Cilag, Lorex Synthelabo, Lundbeck, Organon, Pharmacia and Upjohn, Pierre-Fabre, Pfizer, Rhone-Poulenc Rorer, Roche, SmithKline Beecham, and Solvay. He has been an expert witness in seven legal actions involving SSRIs.

SECTION 2
Prozac and American Culture

LAUREN SLATER

Kafka's Boys
A Story of Sex and Serotonin

Once, sex addicts were treated by priests and shamans, with pillories and guillotines and gleaming clamps to crush the testicles; but what used to be a moral problem is now a medical one, and this is no surprise. Our understanding of sexual compulsion has followed the same trajectory as our understanding of melancholy and moodiness. It is all in the brain, in a series of neural circuits lit to scarlet, guzzling great quantities of tasty chemicals. Goodbye heart, goodbye crotch: voilà the rumpled organ crammed in its sheath of skull. New scientific theories are shedding an interesting light on the biochemistry of perversion and maybe, by extension, on the chemistry of kinkiness, what you and I do, volitionally and consensually, behind closed bedroom doors.

His name, in all seriousness, is Dr. Kafka. He says he cannot rule out a family relation to Franz, though, by the look of it, there is little physical similarity. Dr. Martin Kafka treats and studies what are clinically known as paraphiliacs at McLean Hospital in Belmont, Massachusetts. Paraphilias are sexual disorders characterized by coercion and urgency—think of exhibitionism, voyeurism, and its kinder cousin, fetishism. Closely related to the paraphilias are what Kafka calls the paraphilia related disorders (PRDs), in common vernacular, sex addiction, whose sufferers may not always be breaking the law but who are driven by a libido so excessive they are helplessly pinned beneath its weight.

Kafka is a world-renowned expert in his field. He comes to work each day dressed in a conservative suit, but he likes to laugh and he likes to eat, insisting, always, that I meet him in the cafeteria, where he dines on Otis Spunkmeyer chocolate chip cookies. "My father was a dentist," he says, biting into a bit of chocolate goo, "and I did two years in dental school before I realized it wasn't for me. I like to say"—and here he smiles—"I went from dental to mental."

His practice currently includes 168 patients, more than three-quarters of whom have what by current cultural standards at least is a wayward, perversely heightened libido. His most serious cases are sexual predators, two of whom have murdered several women; his "lite" cases include the old standbys of masculine misery: compulsive porn watchers, compulsive purchasers of prostitutes, and men incapable of monogamy. In the middle range, which makes up the bulk of his caseload, are the guys we often call creeps—the one who peers in your window as you take off your blue bathrobe or who sits next to you on the train and casually traces his thumb over the arc of your breast. He is the man in the red raincoat; you know, you were coming home, carrying your bag of navel oranges, and he let loose, prying apart the slicker's flaps and showing you his glory, and you rushed on, heart pounding. Those, all of them, are Kafka's men.

Kafka did not start out his career focusing on sexual impulse disorders. Oddly, he began by working with women in inpatient units who carried a diagnosis of eating disorders, women so thin the bones rose in ridges through their skin or their throats were chafed from the thrust of their rigid fingers. "One day," says Kafka, "two sex offenders came on the unit. There were no other beds in the hospital, maybe, so they put these guys on the eating disorders unit, and that's when I had my eureka moment. I began to see that the sex offenders were just like the anorexics, the bulimics. Both groups were suffering from a disregulation of appetite. I began to think that paraphilias and the PRDs are to men what eating disorders are to women. I was so excited by this breakthrough I didn't sleep for two nights."

In fact, there are interesting inverse relationships between eating disorders and sexual impulse disorders. The sex distribution of individuals who suffer from paraphilias and PRDs is 95 percent men and 5 percent women, whereas the sex distribution for those with eating disorders is 95 percent women and 5 percent men. Both disorders involve difficulty experiencing satiation as well as a disregulation in appetite drives. Kafka thought he was on to something, and maybe he was. Perhaps he has found the male bulimic, a man who is not bingeing on chocolate but on flesh.

"TSO," says Kafka, "total sexual outlet." We are sitting in his office, which, like his name, is disconcertingly appropriate to his task. His office is in a basement. It is damp, and a dehumidifier luridly gurgles in a corner. "It'd be nice to have bigger windows," he says, "you know?"

"So," he says, "you have to look at total sexual outlet as one way

LAUREN SLATER

of diagnosing a paraphiliac or a PRD. How many times does he masturbate a week? What are the number of orgasms he has per week? Anything over six and my ears perk up."

"Six?" I say. I am surprised by how low the number is. By this definition, my husband may be in trouble.

"What's the average amount a man masturbates?" I say.

"Three," he says. "It varies."

"There must be a lot of paraphiliacs out there that we don't know about," I say.

"There probably are," he says. "In one study, 75 percent of normal men admitted to regular rape fantasies. In another study, penile tumescence between normal men and convicted pedophiles were compared when both groups were shown pornographic pictures of children, and tumescence was just about equal."

I look to my left. On a small glass table, Kafka, a jokester at heart, has his own fake pharmacy. There are medication bottles—red, green, and piglet pink. One has Virginity Restorer, Extra Strength, Cherry Flavored, written in frilly script across the label. There is another bottle called Willpower and a third labeled Passion Control Pills. Kafka sees me staring. "You have to have some humor in my line of work," he says. I nod. I try to imagine the porn addict, the exhibitionist, or the rapist sitting in the seat I occupy now, confessing. I wonder if they think the pills are funny. I wonder if they ever take them—from desperation, desire, or the wish for an easy cure—and feel the sweet sugar in their mouths.

"Sex," says Kafka, "can be a curse."

We have heard, of late, so much about sex and hormones: testosterone, suspended in a golden hue, shot slowly into layered, striated muscle; estrogen rubbed on labial skin, restoring oiliness and glow. One of Kafka's most significant contributions to the chemistry of perversity may be that he has been able to look beyond the obvious culprits—sex steroids—to the more nuanced chemical messengers and the complex roles they play in mediating our desires.

Here is a significant study: There are rats in cages. A scientist lowers his latex-gloved hand, syringe professionally poised, and shoots the mammal up with parachlorophenylalanine (PCA), which lowers serotonin in both blood and brain. Within minutes of its administration there is a steep falloff, a veritable drought of serotonin, and what happens to the rats? They get horny. They mount each other compulsively. Conversely, feed these same rats a serotonin-laced snack, thereby raising their blood levels, and almost all sexual appetite disappears.[1] "In other words," says Kafka, "this isn't just about testosterone. It used to be thought sexual deviants had just testosterone abnormalities, but they may really have serotonin abnormalities. It may be that the lower the serotonin the higher the sex drive, or it may be something much more complex, that sexual deviance is linked to an as yet unidentified disregulation in the serotonin system." Other studies bear this hypothesis out. A male, prior to copulation, has a decrease in serotonin. Post copulation, when he is smoking his cigarette or snoring like he had just chowed down on a turkey dinner, his serotonin levels have soared. In a culture in love with the idea of "high" serotonin, it might surprise us to know that passion and its distant cousin, lewdness, may lie not in the dosed-up but the dosed-down version of being.

Kafka calls his theory of sexual impulse disorders the monoamine hypothesis because he is looking at, and honoring, the central role our monoamines—dopamine, norepinephrine, and specifically, serotonin—play in mediating desire. One of the more interesting studies he cites involves castrated rats that were injected with PCA, which depletes central nervous system serotonin, and that subsequently were able to resume normal mounting behavior *without* any testosterone additives.[2] In other words, at least as far as animal analogues go, serotonin deprivation and its hypothesized partner, depression, appear to be powerful aphrodisiacs.

After hearing Kafka talk about this—after hearing, yet again, about serotonin grabbing the star role in still another psychiatric drama—I asked my husband, a chemist, to bring some of this mysterious chemical home for me, just so I could finally wrap my hands around it. He did, presenting me with a tiny glass tube with WARNING written all over the pasted label: CENTRAL NERVOUS SYSTEM IRRITANT. FOR RDR USE ONLY. I peered inside and was surprised by what I saw. I had always imagined a neurotransmitter would be liquid. How else does it spurt from one ravenous cell to the next? But the serotonin my husband presented me with was crystallized, like salt or snowflakes, and it was talcum to the touch. Beneath our microscope serotonin pulsed into view, six pronged, simplistic as a star. You could cap your Christmas tree with it. Seeing serotonin there, etched out, magnified and crude, it was difficult to believe its presence or absence could cause such a ruckus in the complex beings that we, as human beings, supposedly are.

LAUREN SLATER

"Our brains," says Lawrence Kirmayer, professor of psychiatry at McGill University, "are such incredibly complex organs, so largely beyond our understanding. It's ridiculous to think that any one chemical causes, or is responsible for this or that. It's patently reductive."

But Kafka is not so sure. "Of course it's complex," he says. "All of these systems are interrelated. Who knows, we might find sexual deviance is related to an as yet undiscovered neurotransmission system. But it's plausible," he says, "to hypothesize that serotonin plays a critical part. Because these men respond so well to drugs like Prozac or other SSRIS, which alter serotonin transmission in the brain, it's reasonable to point to that monoamine as central, and maybe even causative in sexual impulse disorders."

That Kafka treats male sexual impulse disorders biologically is nothing new. Castration, which is nothing if not a biological treatment, was used on a "prevert" in 1498 when Gus Rameria, an intractable pedophile, had his testicles crushed by stones cupped in the hands of an angry crowd. If you think that is awfully old-fashioned, it is not. More than 600 elective castrations are performed in the United States annually by men who wish to lower their wayward libidos. The operation, performed primarily by a ghoulish-looking Felix Spector, D.O., in Philadelphia, costs $2,000, takes about eight minutes, and according to one recipient, has postsurgery pain equivalent to "a tooth ache between the thighs."[3]

But Kafka, of course, does not want to castrate his patients. Nor does he want to engage in what is commonly called chemical castration, which amounts to the administration of antiandrogens, testosterone-suppressing compounds that eradicate all sexual desire. What Kafka aims to do by way of treatment is far nobler, far more complex, and far more chemically questionable. He aims, through the use of serotonin selective drugs, to whitewash deviance but somehow spare conventional sexuality, so that the patient, posttreatment, is capable of "affiliative sex" but not bizarreness.

This is an important point, perhaps even the crux of the matter. Drugs like Prozac and Paxil have been hailed for their supposed selectivity. They selectively target the serotonin systems, thereby sparing patients of the widespread side effects of the older generations of antidepressants. But in Kafka's conceptualization, selectivity has reached new heights. Kafka claims that the drugs are somehow selective not only for serotonin systems but for, well, sexual systems, reducing or eradicating one form of desire while preserving or enhancing another. How can this be? Does deviant or dysfunctional lust reside in one part of our brain, and affiliative, conventional lust in another? Is a man's erection when he fetishizes powered by, say, the pituitary, while when he makes love, some other, friendlier lobe raises the tumescent tissue? "Are you sure?" I say to Kafka; "You give a man with sexual problems Prozac and his deviance disappears while his affiliative sexuality emerges?"

"I've seen it happen," says Kafka, "over and over again."

I am curious. I am skeptical. I want to see this in action.

Bill Morrel is not a handsome man. This is the first thing he says to me after he shakes my hand. "I am not a handsome man," he states, lowering his bulky body into the too-small seat across from me, fingers gripping the sides.

"I'm nervous," he says, "and when I'm nervous my nose twitches," which it does, while he snuffs and dabs with a huge splotched hankie.

Bill is fifty-two years old. He wears square glasses, and his jowly face is in need of a shave. No, he is not handsome, but neither is he ugly. In fact, there is something frankly appealing about this man—his palpable anxiety, his willingness to talk. "People need to know," he says. "Go ahead, use my name, use my story, this is a sickness and people need to know, but god, I'm nervous to tell you." Twitch twitch. He touches his throat, as though to take measure of his pulse, which, I imagine, is bebopping at a rate too rapid for his comfort. "All right," he says, "this is what I did."

Bill is a carnival man. He makes $200,000 a year setting up and then disassembling the gear of other peoples' pleasure: painted carousels with plastic golden horses kicking their hooves high in the air, Ferris wheels that jingle and sway, and moonwalks that children bounce on. He is a hard worker, rising at 5:00 A.M. to get the Ferris wheel and cotton candy in order and staying on-site until darkness descends and the first stars appear in the sky.

The carnival grounds where Bill works are full of women: blonds toting plump toddlers around, brunettes opening their painted mouths for spun sugar on gaily striped cones. "I felt my first wave," says Bill, "when I was in my thirties." It came on slowly, a clenching, nervous energy in the stomach, "and then I was totally out of control. I *had* to have a woman."

The waves, the waves. Bill talks at length about the waves, their slow or sudden build, their muscular thrusts, how consuming they were, a total corporeal takeover that resulted in his picking up prostitutes, cruising for hours on end, woman after woman in a Dionysian but dystonic frenzy, Ambers and Jo Jos and Mandys and Sunshines all in a pool of semen and pulse. "Exhausting," says Bill. "And I'm married. All this time, through all these women, I was married."

Prior to treatment, Bill describes a life of crippling sexual obsession, a life where he was driven, day after day after miserable day, to exhausting and exhibitionistic bouts of intercourse in bus stations, in front of city halls, in the backseats of Greyhounds, in elevators with the STOP button engaged, on sidewalks in the half-hidden shade in the high heat of summer. He describes sitting at the dinner table with his wife and feeling himself jerked upward by a powerful, invisible hand, reeling out into the night, leaving behind him a thick trail of lies. "I never got anything done," he says. "I was totally unreliable. Sex was to me what sleep was to a narcoleptic. I was in horror of it. Desire would come on. I'd drop down and wake up and have lost a whole day, who knows. I lost twenty years of my life."

In addition to the bars and the highways and all those public places, Bill was driven to masturbate four or five times daily. "Sound impossible?" he says. "It's not." In the mornings after getting up, he had to watch at least one hour of porn, and ditto in the evening before bed. "But it was mostly the waves," he says. "I could get them anywhere. I kept a mattress in the back of my van just so I could get a prostitute as quick as possible. My van has more mileage inside than out."

At first, Bill thought he was simply oversexed. "But then I noticed," he says, "that in my forties the waves started coming more and more. They were especially bad after rainstorms."

"And did your wife know about this behavior?" I asked him.

"Oh no," he says.

"Did you have sex with your wife as well?" I ask.

"Sure," he says.

"Was it good sex?" I ask.

"It was okay," he says, "but not forbidden. Married sex is vanilla. I needed something dangerous. Anne, though, my wife, she's a super person. A super person. She's a Gemini. I'm a Sagittarius. We just blend."

Finally, at age fifty, Bill succumbed to what he feels is the vilest deed: repeated sex with an adolescent neighbor, and one, no less, who had spent her formative years playing in his house.

"I was in a wave," Bill said, "which is why it happened with Kelly. She was so *young*. You've gotta understand. In a wave, anything can be sexual to me." He points to the lamp on the desk. "Like that lamp," he says. "In a wave that lamp could turn me on."

Dr. Peter Martin of Vanderbilt University Addictions Treatment Center elucidates. Using functional MRI scans, Martin, along with his colleague Dr. Paul Regan, is in the initial stages of studying the parts of the brain involved in arousal. "If we can classify what parts of the brain are involved in normal arousal," he says, "then maybe we can see if these parts are different in normal volunteers versus men with sexual addictions or paraphilias," he says. He explains his own hunch to me. He tells me he thinks that "sex addicts" or sex offenders might show activation in a larger portion of the brain than a normal volunteer would in response to a stimulus. In other words, Martin hypothesizes that men with sexual impulse disorders might have a more generalized response, whereas arousal in a more normal person would be fixed in a particular cerebral spot. On an MRI, the aroused paraphiliac brain might look like a veritable lobe of livid florescence, whereas the aroused normal brain might look like, well, a normal brain, a gray, moth-shaped thing with a little point of turquoise excitation. If this proves to be true, then in men like Bill sex may bleed into the brain's more general geography, and thus such brains may be more capable than the rest of turning everyday, commonplace events, and even objects, into erotic tools. Bill's brain, perhaps, can make an aluminum lamp from Staples into some lithe and fluid fantasy object, whereas my brain is, in some sense, far less plastic. The lamp stays in the lamp slot, and the lamp slot is not the sex slot; I am straight, very straight. Bill blurs and blends.

Perhaps.

In any case, I reach over and switch off the lamp. Bill laughs. "I like you," he says. "I feel you're on my side. Now, before treatment, if I had feelings of liking you, they'd go elsewhere. I'm not a handsome man, but before treatment I was so out of control, and I could get any woman. I wouldn't be afraid to say, 'I'll give you a thousand dollars to bend over.' And who knows, you might do it."

I shrug. Bill, by the way, is the seventh man I have interviewed for this story. All the patients I talk to claim to be more or less cured, but all of them spike their conversation with troublesome, inverted kinds of come-ons that at first made me uncomfortable and that now, well, trigger little reaction. I wonder if I am getting numb. Say sex enough times and it starts to sound like x x x x, which is not porn but nothing, nowhere, zero, dead. What the victims sometimes are.

"Well," I say, "I don't know about that."

"I tried to kill myself," he says, "after the Kelly incident."

I nod.

"I lit my trailer on fire, with me in it. When that didn't work, I decided to jump off the crane in the Quincy shipyard. It's called a Goliath Crane, 380 feet tall, the tallest crane in North America; it can pick up 1,300 tons, which is just enough to pick up my mother-in-law on a good day."

Bill laughs. I laugh. Bill is a successful sex addict but an unsuccessful suicide. The pulse beats in his throat. The blood filters in and out of his generous, bendable brain. He went through fire and rain, shocked himself on a live wire, leaped into the air, pulled downward by the weight of his own sweaty hulk, and he is still here today to tell it. He survived his suicide attempts and, upon waking up each time to find the breath still in his body, decided maybe he could kill a part of himself instead of the whole package. "I went to a doctor at Mass. General and told them to take care of it." He points to his groin. "Cut it off. Kill it. No doc would touch me."

Bill finally found his way to Kafka's basement on the gracious grounds of McLean. He sat across from Kafka and talked. "Kafka is a great man. He knew just what questions to ask. I filled out a million questionnaires. He looked at them and said, 'I think I know what's wrong with you. You are a sexual compulsive.'"

Kafka treated Bill solely with medications. "What about psychotherapy?" I ask Kafka. "Don't these guys have a problem in their pasts?"

Common wisdom has it that the sexually compulsive themselves were often victims of sexual abuse, and, thus, their present behavior is interpreted as a kind of repetition compulsion. "The fact is," says Kafka, "only one-quarter to one-third of my patient population suffered physical or sexual abuse, and many of them had unremarkable childhoods, as far as I can see." So, we are back to the start, the tip of the iceberg, the top of the body—the brain. Where it all begins.

Kafka is not a shy man. How could he be? He traffics in semen and blood. He went from dental to mental and is not afraid to say it. At lectures, which he often gives, he says to the audience, "Okay, now I'm going to show you a close-up picture of the male sex organ. I know that's not orthodox, to show sex organs at lectures, so those of you who are uncomfortable, feel free to leave."

Of course no one leaves. The audience inevitably grows hushed, breathless, waiting to see what they see every night, in the shower, on the sheets, endlessly mundane and endlessly fascinating. Kafka flips to the slide. Up on the sparkling white screen a huge brain glows, and down beneath this sprightly little man gleefully points. "The male sex organ," he proudly announces to guffaws and applause; he always gets, as he puts it, a rise.

This is why he treats his men with pills, not talk. In Bill's case the pill was not Prozac but Celexa, a newer version of pretty much the same stuff. Here comes the common part of the story. Bill went home and swallowed a pill. Then he swallowed a second pill. Kaboom. There goes Jekyll. Here comes Hyde. Or is it the other way around? Bill #1 melted away and Bill #2 stepped forward. "On these pills," says Bill, "I am a different man. My head is clear as a bell. I can go with the flow. But the weirdest thing is," he says, and here his voice drops in wonder, "the weirdest thing is how huggy I am now. I was never a huggy person before. I was always afraid I'd want more. But now I hug people left and right. I'll hug people I haven't seen in twenty years. This medication has turned me into a man who likes to hug."

Bill leans forward. For one treacherous moment I think he is going to hug me, but, thankfully, he collapses back, exhaling his astonishment. "Really it's quite amazing," he says.

"So you don't excessively masturbate or do porn or sleep with prostitutes or have intercourse in the backs of buses on a regular basis anymore," I say.

"No more," he says. "I have no urge."

Okay. Here is the part I am interested in. "What about your wife," I say. "How's sex with her?" I have been waiting awhile to get here, to see how "affiliative sex" perseveres or, in Bill's case, burgeons, in the face of this chemical assault, as Kafka has told me it does.

"Listen," he says, "sex is dead. It's dead," he says, briefly patting his crotch like it is a pet. "It's gone."

"So you don't have sex with your wife either?" I say.

"Only when she insists," he says. "And then, I'm good for maybe a minute, if at all."

"I see," I say, but I do not.

Prozac and its chemical cousins have been hailed as so many things: antidepressants, anxiolytics, smoking cessation agents, PMS drugs, shyness drugs, back pain drugs. Here is a new use for them, as far as I can tell: chemical castrators. Kafka does not like this idea, as it flies directly in the face of his pioneering effort, which is to restore normal sex drive while wiping out deviance. But Bill points to another

LAUREN SLATER

possibility. The SSRIs work in the treatment of paraphiliacs and sex addicts because—and everyone knows this—they dampen if not destroy libido, along with all sorts of other excessive behaviors. This is a far less lyrical and exciting conceptualization than the idea of separate sexual systems linked one to the conventional, the other to the crude, but it makes more intuitive, if not scientific, sense. Who knows; one day Prozac may be approved for chemical castration, or some toned-down version of such.

Kafka strongly reacts to this suggestion on my part. I do not want to hurt his feelings or throw a wrench into his theories, but, well, evidence is evidence. The SSRIs cause sexual dysfunction in 80 percent of users, so why not use them to impair an overly functioning man? "Sexual dysfunction," says Kafka, "is *not* the same as chemical castration. These men *can* function sexually, it's just sometimes difficult. Furthermore, chemical castration came out of a need to punish these guys whereas my aim is to help and value these men."

Now that is an interesting response. Pharmacology, like crime, can be judged not only by outcome but by intent. If you did not intend to murder the person, then it is manslaughter. If you do not intend to castrate the person, then it is . . . what? But Kafka has a point. You cannot easily tease apart the cure from the cure giver; medicine is an amalgam of hopes, intentions, and observable results. The placebo effect underscores this. The drug is inextricably bound up with the patient's expectations. In Kafka's scheme, the doctor's expectations get thrown into the mix, as well they should. A drug is as much a wish as a fact.

All philosophizing aside, Bill is happy, actually gleeful with his outcome. "It's dead and I love it," he crows. I add this for a purpose. He is not the first man to bow down in gratefulness to his ruined sexuality. Many sex addicts and sex offenders hate their sexuality. They see it as "the devil." It is alien, horrific to the humane sides of their personality, which are everywhere in evidence. Bill holds hands with his wife and walks on the beach. Keith, a pedophile, is an artist who lovingly designs houses and pots. Bob, an exhibitionist, takes pride in his brand new Hyundai, polishing its black armor until it shines healthy as onyx. Kind men. Careful men. "Sick men we are," says Bill.

"But *not* castrated," says Kafka, whose delicate hands are steepled in front of his face as we talk. "Go ahead, call Bill and ask him if he feels I've castrated him, if he feels he's been castrated by my treatment."

So I do. Two weeks after our initial interview, I do.

"Do you feel you've been castrated?" I say to Bill over the phone.

"Of course," he says, "and Kafka's the only doc who had the balls to do it."

Why or how Prozac blunts sexuality is open to speculation. Animal studies clearly show a correlation between raised or altered serotonin and diminished sexual appetite. In addition, both serotonin and dopamine do an intricate dance with our hormones, priming neural pathways so they can respond to testosterone. "I don't think," says Peter Martin, "that the SSRIs are really capable of restoring a normal sex drive. We all know that the SSRIs cause sexual dysfunction. The sex addict or the 'overly sexed' man may have such a large portion of his brain dedicated to arousal that a blunted sex drive just looks like a normal sex drive, which is much different than the idea of two separate sexual systems, one for deviance, one for love."

Here is Vinny. He is one of Kafka's star patients. "You have to talk to Vinny," he says. "Vinny has such a good outcome." Kafka leaves two messages on my machine to make sure I have contacted Vinny. He is like a parent, proud of his boy. "Vinny is evidence," he says, "of how a paraphiliac can take medication and become sexually normal. He is fully functional."

"But *why* is he functional?" I ask. "Is he blunted, or has something been restored?"

Kafka sighs. He is probably tired of my questions. Yet this distinction is important to me. If the SSRIs cure a man by inducing sexual dysfunction, then they are in some essential sense not normalizing eroticism but just transmogrifying it in yet a new way. Is this the role of good medicine, to cure one illness by inducing another? Is this medicine or iatrogenic injury? Maybe, especially in the case of dangerous predators, a little injury is healing. But let's call a spade a spade. Replacing one dysfunction with another is problematic practice and is certainly different from treating a person with drugs that restore the flesh to its rightful homeostasis.

Vinny is definitive, sure of himself, free of Bill's twitches and tics. He is an insurance agent and works clean columns of numbers eight hours a day. His nails are buffed pale sunrises below trimmed cuticles. His dress is impeccable: pressed chinos, a red Ferrari shirt, a gold linked bracelet and one gold chain, "straight from Italy," he says, a cross and his grandmother's pendant dangling on his massive chest.

Vinny's DSM diagnosis is 313.00, transvestic fetishism. He grew up in a traditional Italian household, the kind with dark curtains hanging

LAUREN SLATER

on the windows and red gravy bubbling on the black-topped stove. He recalls his father with anger, a distant, towering man, quick with his whipping words, and his mother and grandmother with untrammeled affection. "My grandmother was a seamstress," he says, "and we visited her every weekend on Powder House Boulevard." There, Vinny learned the luxury of textiles, the hum of the Singer sewing machine, and the metamorphosis of crushed red velvet and rhinestones into cocktail dresses. "She made clothes for my mother and aunts," he says, "and I used to see my mother swoosh out in her new gowns and I'd say, 'Mom, you look GORGEOUS.'"

He was eight years old when his problem began, a terrible burning secret that grew as the years went by. He started, in secret, to try on his mother's clothes. This gave him such a soothing thrill, "the silky parts against my privates," that it burgeoned into a full-blown compulsion culminating each time in an act of masturbation into his mother's underwear. He engaged in this repetitive ritualistic behavior until he was twenty-six years old, always with his mother's garments. "I liked her thigh-high stockings," he says. "I liked her black silk panties and her slips and her teddies."

At twenty-seven, Vinny moved out of his mother's house to get married. His wife knew nothing of his behavior. "Now it was really terrible," he says, "because we had this two-bedroom apartment and I bought all these clothes from Frederick's of Hollywood catalogs or from Sears, and I had to hide them in this really small space. And I spent too much money at Saugus Shoe Town buying thigh-high boots. I was so afraid she'd find out. Still, I'd cross-dress whenever I got the chance, when she was in the shower, when she was at work, when she was asleep. And I began, also, to be cruel to her. I'd force her into sex acts. This put a damper between us."

Vinny describes a life of tortured fashion—a life of sordidness not necessarily because it *is* sordid (although it is hard to interpret spousal force as anything except that), but because he experienced the fetished cross-dressing that way, partly for cultural reasons, of course. "Look," he says, "I'm not gay. I never wore makeup. Okay?"

"But don't you think," I say, "that if the culture condoned this kind of behavior, it wouldn't have been so problematic for you? It wouldn't have grown so compulsive? Maybe it was the shame that made it a problem."

"No," says Vinny. He says this swiftly, dicing my words right down. "I sometimes think what would have happened if I went out with this.

Went onto the streets like some men do. With free reign, my problem would have gotten worse and worse and worse until my whole self was lost. I would have been nothing but cloth."

One night, two years into his marriage, after a particularly compulsive day of cross-dressing that left him demoralized and exhausted, Vinny had a vivid dream. His car crashed and flew weightless as an angel over a cliff, with him inside. He was not, in the dream, afraid of dying, but afraid of what would happen when his wife went through his possessions and found his secret stash of ostrich plumes and slingback pumps and monstrous teddies.

He woke up soaked not in semen but in sweat. His wife lay curled on her side, away from him, "an object," he says, "someone to fuck. Not a person. But I always loved her anyway." He resolved to change after that dream.

He started treatment with Carol Ball, Ph.D., at the New England Forensic Institute in Arlington, Massachusetts. Treatment with paraphiliacs follows a fairly predictable pattern. Men describe what is called systematic desensitization. They are instructed to masturbate to a deviant fantasy and at the point of climax to breathe deeply of ammonia, only to come in a clutch of coughs and cramps. Another standard behavioral treatment technique is called orgasm reconditioning, wherein the man masturbates to his deviant fantasy, ejaculates, and then continues to masturbate past the point of pleasure. Yet another technique involves willfully substituting a "normal" fantasy for a deviant one earlier and earlier in the masturbatory sequence. The exterior of the New England Forensic Institute belies the gruesome and bizarre training techniques taking place within its walls. A building painted chirpy yellow, with pots of mums beaming on its stoop, it welcomes.

Behavioral therapy with sexual impulse disorders is highly successful. Some judges will even mandate less dangerous men to the institute instead of to jail. Two months after Vinny went to the institute, Carol Ball referred him to Dr. Kafka for a medication consult. "Behavioral treatment is very effective," says Ball, "but we still refer 99 percent of our men for medication, because of comorbidity, and because treatment works best in combination."

Vinny credits Kafka, not Ball, with the bulk of his success. "I love Carol Ball," he says. "But it was the medication, definitely the medication that really changed things for me."

Kafka put Vinny on what appears to be his fairly standard drug fare, the newer SSRI, Celexa. "Within three months I felt totally different,"

Vinny says. "All my cross-dressing urges were gone. The shoe fetish was gone. I put the teddies, the Frederick's of Hollywood stuff, the panties, the thigh-highs—I put it all in a duffel bag and threw it in the dumpster. It was just like closing a closet door."

Vinny reports that he has no more urges to cross-dress, no more consuming fetishes, and no more desires to force his wife into daily or twice-daily sex. He has not masturbated since he began drug treatment. "My life in the past eleven months has been better than it's been in the past twenty-eight years," he says. "I have possibilities."

The difference between Vinny and Bill Morrel is that Vinny enjoys what sounds to be a very normal sex life with his wife. "Three times a week," he says. "I have no trouble. My orgasms are actually better on the Celexa than they were off. It's because on the Celexa I can really concentrate on my wife's body and not on the fantasies and fetishes, which before interfered. Crystal, my wife, is gorgeous. She's petite, five three, one hundred and ten pounds. I can relax into her. We take our time. We are very relaxed now."

He describes his recovery in still more detail. "The fetishisms," he says, "were like all this static. Now the static's cleared away and what's left is my real desire. My head feels like a whole new thing. My real desire is not for my mother or for a man, but for my wife. Crystal is my temple."

Of course it is evident why Kafka wanted me to meet Vinny. He is a poster boy for successful treatment outcomes. He is living, walking proof that at least some men experience not a preferable form of dysfunction but an erotic restoration under Kafka's care. If, in fact, drugs like Prozac and Celexa can selectively wipe out deviance while restoring or even enhancing "normal" sexuality, what might this mean about the way our brains are built?

In the 1980s, neuroscientists made a series of fascinating discoveries. One stroke victim who suffered lesions to his left parietal lobe could recall all of the names of fruits but none of the names of flowers. Other amnesiac patients recalled with ease all canine breeds, but felines had melted into the mist. This raised the possibility that our brains are modular and store information in category-specific locales that can be deleted with the simple burst of a bright blood vessel. This modular notion of brain function appears to expand beyond the domain of language recall. Daniel Schacter, Larry R. Squire, and Michael Posner, among other neuroscientists, have written extensively about separate memory systems with separate neural substrates: short term versus long term, declarative versus implicit, and motor memory versus word-based recall. Why, then, might not forms of sexual appetite or desire be divided as well? Patients with brain tumors in the temporo-limbic system sometimes experience not only a marked increase in sex drive but a change in sexual preference as well. People who develop seizure disorders, which are often linked to lesions in a very specific part of the brain, may also display exhibitionistic behavior. There is a very rare disorder called Kluver Bucy Syndrome in which the amygdala is damaged and the patient experiences intense sexual desire for objects such as pins, cups, and who knows, maybe even lamps. Patients with Kluver Bucy Syndrome will also often develop transvestism. Perhaps in an effort to illuminate some of the mysteries of all this, a few years ago French scientists put a "normal" couple into an MRI scanner, where they made love in the hum of deep magnets. Does Vinny's brain look different when he makes love to Crystal than when he is in the act of orgasming in thigh-highs—the amygdala versus the striatum, perhaps, or the limbic versus the frontal lobe? Or have we fallen, once again, into relentless reductionism?

Kafka does not know, and he is not afraid to say so. "But it *is* interesting to speculate," he says, "that normal male sexual arousal resides in one area of the brain, deviant sexual arousal in another, and that the ssris work by targeting one arousal system while sparing another. That's an interesting, plausible hypothesis, and one that wouldn't surprise me."

Another possibility is this: the higher the intensity of any drive, the more polymorphous its manifestations. The ssris may work in paraphilias and sexual addiction not by deleting but more simply by pruning so that the person's core sexuality is free to finally emerge. This hypothesis may lie most closely to the idea some psychiatrists hold: that the paraphilias are simply another form of obsessive-compulsive disorder, and that the ssris work not because they target sexual arousal but because they are known to reduce ruminative thoughts and repetitive behaviors in all kinds of conditions. "I hate that idea," says Kafka. "The paraphilias and PRDs are not a form of OCD [obsessive-compulsive disorder]. People who have OCD do not have an appetite disregulation disorder. OCD is not about appetite. Sexual impulse disorders are *all* about appetite."

Oh well. In the end, your head just swims with all the speculation. Where, oh where, I wonder, is speculation located in the brain? I can tell you. It is three inches up from the cerebellum, a little left of the thrumming thalamus, right where my headache is just, this moment, starting to hammer away.

What, after all of this, can I offer you by way of fact? On one hand, nothing. On the other hand, something. We have these men; they are facts. That they feel better is a fact. That Prozac and its chemical cousins have yet another use is a fact. That its uses are so widespread as to present us with a boggling contradiction is a fact. Here we have a drug celebrated for its specificity but employed for every nook and cranny of our multiple miseries; that, surely, is a fact. The rats are a fact—their serotonin-starved brains, their tails luridly atwitch. That when we think of sex or brains or love or deviance we are reflexively reductive is also a troublesome fact. "Please," says my friend and literary critic Harvey Blume when I read him a portion of this story, "please don't tell me about another reductive Prozac-pushing doctor. Doesn't this guy believe in history? In society?"

Of course he does. First of all, Kafka is doing something very right. He has "cured," or restored to better balance, more than 600 men, many of whom are dangerous and all of whom are, by their own standards at least, terribly twisted. Kafka's patients love him. "He is THE GUY," says Jim B. "He saved my life," says Bob R. "But where," says Harvey Blume, "where is the history, the culture in this story. No more neurospeak, okay?"

Kafka, obviously, practices neurospeak; but oddly enough, if you are looking for culture, you will find it right where he dwells, in that basement office, above the Passion Control Pills. On my last visit to Kafka I notice what I have oddly not noticed in all my visits before: large and very beautiful photographs on almost every inch of wall space seem to gleam in the low light. "I took these pictures myself," says Kafka when I ask. He has traveled all over the world. Here, above me, a Peruvian boy holds his little naked brother, fat dimpled buttocks, a sweet grin. Across the way, Italian women play cards beneath flags of laundry on a line; the photo is shot in saturated yellow light, the fabric as human as flesh, vivid, living. I walk around the room, staring in appreciation. There are photos taken in the Himalayas, in Poland, in Timbuktu. There is a photo of a zebra, an extreme close-up of the animal's face, the dark, dilated eye with wisps of tangled lashes. I am looking into the zebra's eye when Kafka's phone rings. I hear him pick it up. "Good," he says. "So you're not doing that anymore? I'm so glad. But the Prozac's working now. Good."

He hangs up, comes to stand next to me. "I took this picture," he says, "at the Kenyan Zoo. The zebra was wounded, in a cage, so I could get real close to him, put the camera right up next to his face, and I got this shot of his eye."

The eye, of course, is a part of our brains, a little bit of the visual cortex poking unsheathed and vulnerable through our flesh. Kafka pulls into himself. I recall how he told me, over lunch a few days ago, that in this line of work he has seen the devil, and the devil has neural substrates, but something more as well. "I have become theistic," he said, and he looked troubled. Then he said, "You know, my patients are my boys. They're all my boys. Have you called my boy, Paul?"

Now Kafka seems to forget I am here. He reaches out and touches his photograph, the eye, this bit of animal brain exposed, unknowable. He touches tenderly, almost sadly, and watching him do this, I have to wonder if it is the proffered pill or his hand held out that, for these men, finally turns the trick.

NOTES

1. See M. P. Kafka, "A Monoamine Hypothesis for the Pathophysiology of Paraphilic Disorders," *Archives of Sexual Behavior* 26 (1997): 337–52. For rat studies, see E. Menendez-Abraham, P. Moran-Viesca, and A. Velasco-Plaxa, "Modifications of the Sexual Activity in Male Rats following the Administration of Serotoninergic Drugs," *Behavior and Brain Research* 30 (1988): 251–58; B. J. Everitt and J. Bancroft, "Of Rats and Men: The Comparative Approach to Male Sexuality," in *Annual Review of Sex Research*, ed. J. Bancroft, C. M. Davis, and H. J. Ruppel Jr. (Mt. Vernon, Iowa: Society for the Scientific Study of Sex, 1991), 77–118.

2. A. Tagliamonte, P. Tagliamonte, and G. L. Gessa, "Compulsive Sexual Activity Induced by P-chlorophenylalanine in Normal and Pinealectomized Rats," *Science* 166 (1969): 1433–35.

3. See <www.felixspector.com>.

LAURIE ZOLOTH

Care of the Dying in America

INTRODUCTION

The Kid

In the late summer of 2000, I returned on a late night flight from a semester teaching in Virginia. It was midmorning before I went out to buy groceries and settle back into my Berkeley neighborhood. It was a startling little trip, because all along the way there were adults skimming along the sidewalks on bright metal scooters, the kind I used to play with as a child. Yellow sunlight was beginning to burn the fog away and gleamed on the baseball caps and the backpacks of the riders. It seemed an odd scene, but a familiar one. It was a picture from my own 1950s childhood: happy gliding children on the scooters, pushing along the wide white suburban sidewalk with rubber-soled sneakers. In the 1950s, we were pretending to be grown-ups in cars, so we made small growly noises in our throats—rum, rum—simulating ignition and vast power. But these were grown-ups now, pretending the opposite—that they were children, and that the adult life they were engaged in was not that at all, but a kind of game that made them happy.

I realized that while I had been away in a place that seemed intensely engaged in the past, in the Jeffersonian rhetoric and the way that the young American colonialists in their twenties had reconfigured and rewritten the world, my city had bounded ever more buoyantly into the next new thing, and that seemed to be a deepening of a flight into childhood as the pursuit of happiness. It was shortly thereafter that Carl Elliott asked me to think about the new pharmaceuticals for depression. He was interested in what ethicists made of how the widespread and thematized use of antidepressant medication, and the idea that depression was a new and metaphoric "epidemic,"[1] had shaped our conceptions of self and hence shaped the culture these altered selves both created and were created by. He knew that I, as an ethicist writing from within the tradition of Jewish moral philosophy, was interested in evil and in moral choice, and he queried whether there was a sense in which thinking of anger or despair as an illness to be treated with a pill, or a chemical imbalance that can be fixed, altered the canon of moral philosophy and shook a core task and telos of its project, the struggle to understand and live a good life.

Thus it has become my theory, in part, that how we are living in this "time of Prozac" is made possible in large part because we are living in a culture of great yearning and great expectation, a culture obsessed with flight from mortal limits and adult burdens. It is a yearning for a time and a place as far as we can get from death. And such a place is an imagined childhood. Thus it is not happiness we seek, exactly, but the relief from the complexities of being. If one can be, rather, a being outside of being, outside of temporality, one could be safe. Being is a difficult and grief-stricken task, because being a being-in-time means you will die. Children who grow into adults grow against and through temporal space and become into being, take on the burden of being, both in the existential sense and in the literal sense—becoming encumbered, carrying the things one needs to complete the work of humans in the world. Adults bear others along: whining and hungry children, ill and confused parents. It is, in a word, a hard row to hoe—tearing the food from the earth by the sweat of our brows. It is the essence of adulthood—knowing good and evil, having serious matters at stake, carrying death into the world, even in the act of love, as we conceive our replacements.

After 9/11

How to think about this problem of despair is the problem of this essay itself—one that ended up being written in, as we all ended up living in, a very different America, a post–September 11 America, a place in which, suddenly, the Great Death from which we were fleeing was graphically, terribly, in front of us, and the grief and despair paralyzed us all. In many ways, this made the flight I described here ever more poignant, and in other ways, it rendered it mute; it turned out that, after all, Americans were capable of the supererogatory acts that adult life requires. Heroes were not only possible, they were everywhere. It was true that Prozac use rose dramatically after the attack. Indeed, the companies were quick to make up little commercials showing worried urban dwellers complaining of "not being able to stop the tape in my head, worrying over and over," or of "always fearing the worst," and were selling the product in this novel way, the subtext of which was clearly to say if one was haunted by images of falling bodies or of orphaned children or of anthrax, even this could be fixed by Prozac. But that it cannot be fixed, that we now turn and face the thing, itself, only intensifies the problem of culture, self, and sorrow and death.

In this essay I undertake three distinct conversations with you, reader, that interrupt one another in different ways. First, I explore the cultural phenomenon of the yearning for childhood that I argue frames our understanding of depression. Second, I explore the limits of this analysis in the face of some examples of clinical depression, challenging the adequacy of my own thesis. Third, I explore alternative ways of thinking about the problem of depression, social anxiety, and despair, especially from Jewish intellectual philosophic traditions. Finally, I turn to traditional Talmudic texts and the contextual community practices that emerge from them to ask if the recovery of such a tradition might offer alternate responses to despair.

PART 1: THE CHILD WITHIN

We are worried and saddened by our finitude, weary of the hard work of becoming an adult, weary of the way a body ages into death, so we want to head out West, only there is no West to go to, only the simulacrum of the West we know from our time with the Lone Ranger and Tonto. We want not only to be happy, but to be in the happy place where nothing is dying and sorrow can be fixed with, say, a Good Humor bar. We want a place—a suburb of the 1950s, a leave-it-to-Beaver sort of place, in which our happiness was a thing assured, in which our silly troubles could be wrapped up in thirty minutes.

As my proof text, let us consider a list:

The Matter of Dressing the Part

More and more, I see adults wearing baseball caps. This occurs at all times and places: at court appearances, at social events, and at work. When I was a child, men and women wore hats, beautiful hats, and one can see this in the movies of the 1940s and 1950s. In fact, in the game in which one played grown-up, one wore one's parents' old hats and gloves. This is a commonplace of literature, as in C. S. Lewis novels and in all the coming-of-age films and narratives: one puts on hats and long pants; one dresses the part.

Today, we are urged into silly clothes. Clothes for social occasions, such as hats and gloves, were the first to go, but next were suits and ties. It began on casual days, as if we were at some sort of camp, but has now extended to so many places that one is hard pressed to find serious clothes, and such things have a discrete section actually called "interview suits," for the last formal moment left to us. On my campus, it has become stylish to wear bib overalls, as if one were a small toddler who could not be annoyed by a belt. In fact, if one wears a suit, for example, one is queried—as if it were an oddity.

Men wear long ponytails, and this is done even if the ponytail area is the only place where the hair is present. Large, elaborate canvas sneakers are worn on all occasions, as if one is about to take off to the playground. In fact, with the casual attire, the whole effect is that of a cheery beach outing with Mom and Dad. Adults wear backpacks, often in expensive fabrics, or student book bags, instead of briefcases. Women's shoe stores widely display a type of shoe that is an exact copy of little girls' shoes called "Mary Janes," the very name reflecting the childhood dress-up quality. They have straps across the top, like the shoes of toddlers. Velcro closures, first used in the shoes of children too young to tie a shoestring into a bow, are increasingly popular on these shoes.

Adults carry small bottles with them at all times, as if they are on a scout hiking trip, and not in a buildings with indoor plumbing and water fountains. These bottles have nipples on them, and of late are fashioned so that they can be gently squeezed, so that people can suck the water out of the little red nipples that are attached to the ends. Once only distributed at gyms, they are now placed at conference tables, so that at business meetings, rows of professional can sit across from one another all clutching their own bottles.

The Syntax of Childhood

Adults commonly speak in the syntax of their youth. Being "pissed off," "being cool," and "being bummed" are terms used not only in common speech but in advertising campaigns directed at adults. In a related linguistic development, words are commonly misspelled to make them easier to deal with, and the misspellings give the entire text the feel of a second-grader's essay (tonite, lite, etc.).

Nomenclature is informal, as if we were children. Presidents are called Bill and Jimmy and Dubya. Waiters introduce themselves by their first names. Even at academic conferences, one is given a name tag with one's first name, and just in case you might not know, the name tag actually tells you "Hello, my name is ———." This is supposed to encourage good playmate behavior. Speech is informal as well, with phrasing, topics, and the disclosure appropriate for recess, as the topic for prime time.

In fact, an entire universe of corporate consultation has emerged in which the "child" within us is encouraged to come out in public business and academic encounters. In this way, one is supposed to be more "authentically" the self, as if a return to childhood was in some way going back to a better self, a freer self, one existing, in Rousseauian manner, prior to the troubling constructions of adult civilization.

It's a Small World after All

The marketing and acquisition of consumer goods, once seen as necessary items for the reproduction of social life, has become commonly referred to as "getting toys." The Skymall catalog, given out in all airplanes, for example, proudly calls itself "the best place for toys," and this does not refer to items for children but for highly sophisticated technology. Take, for example, a recent ad for an electronics store, in which a woman in her thirties is speaking to a man one presumes is her thirty-year-old husband. She tells him firmly that they are only going to the store for some necessities, in and out. He agrees, but when they get there, he is unable to contain his urges and, quite literally, runs childlike, a little crookedly, away, while she screams his name after him—"Kevin! Come back here!" This confusion about who is the baby and who is the parent is manifest in another commercial in which a grown man is pushing a shopping cart with a baby in it. The baby is pointing at toys and saying "ooh," and the man turns away again and again from the baby's desire. But then they turn a corner, and a car, made up to look as if it were a toy in the store, is on display; for this they stop, and the man says "ooh." In another commercial, the camera flips between a boy riding a bike and a man driving a sports car of great price, while the breathless voice of the advertiser tells us to "remember that feeling!" The sports car, it is suggested, will have a transformative power; one will become the boy on the bike—the final cut is of the boy flying through the air on his bike, evocative of yet another culture reference, that of the savior boys in the film *E.T.* riding to the rescue of mankind over the objections of adult scientists.[2]

Cars are the stand-in for the language of desire—but it is childish desire. Cars, in this syntax (understood as toys), are designed to deny their true use in the world of work or family life as basically a big cart. "Station wagon" bespeaks of family and obligation, but "sport utility vehicle" is a different matter. It is the car of the National Geographic Society explorer, calling to mind Kiplingesque pretend games in which one wears a pith helmet and carries a fake gun. Other cars emerge that are themselves little parodies of cars of the past—reissued Volkswagen "beetles" and "PT cruisers," which look precisely like the rounded toys of children, without harmful edges.

In another ad, the confusion about who the child is and who the adult is, and who takes care of whom, deepens disturbingly: a grown man, a father, wants a glass of milk but has neglected to go to the store, and his desire for milk is so intense that the man steals the last available milk from his own baby's bottle.

In another ad, it is not only parents but teachers and officials who cannot be trusted. An entire Disneyland campaign rests on this theme: There is a spelling bee, and an earnest child, who begins to spell a word "M-I-C," is interrupted (her childhood metaphorically interrupted) by the chorus of adult judges who push her aside to chant "MIC-KEY-MOUSE!" Then they are seen at Disneyland, in their gray hair and suits, on the rides, playing like children, without the actual child. You are never too old to return to Disneyland!

In several ads, cars or computers are the new expensive toys that any boy or girl really wants. The issue of possession as a kind of "toy," as in the phrase "he who dies with the most toys wins," means that the idea of work as a craft or skill that one trains for is less important than the acquisition of the paycheck at the end of the day, since what matters is the toy-commodity. Here, the self is prefigured as a child, the one who yearns for toys, and not the parent, the one who might work and then acquire necessities for a family. Linked to this is the idea that such goods are really more like toys—breakable, replaceable, and not real—and not items of craft, made by adults to be used by adults and handed down to children across generations, such as a fine tool. Toys last a few years at best; one becomes bored and moves on.

Nostalgia and Veracity

Popular culture has taken on an ironic stance. But behind the self-mockery of modern advertising, there lies some truth. The very ads of the 1950s are recycled and seen as adorable, chic, and funny, but they are also relying on the message of all nostalgia—that the past is more authentic, more real, and more trustworthy than the present. It is also true that if one witnesses the very ad style of the 1950s, one is subliminally drawn into the child self of that era.

The nostalgia for the 1950s and 1960s goes beyond ads. In fact, the very clothes are being rereleased, with homage to the 1960s in prints and styles. Bell-bottom pants and platform shoes are in style, as is oldies music. Retro-glasses, as if one were in the fifth grade in 1962, are commonly worn. Articles on food rehearse the theme that veracity, happiness, and authenticity are to be found in childhood delights. There is a genre of food called comfort food, and by this one means the soft baby food of childhood, such as mashed potatoes, as if one did not yet have teeth or was still wary of complex spices or colors.

In movies, we have been treated to two powerful genres that confirm my theory. First, and most simply, there are constant remakes and rehearsals of the popular culture of the 1950s and 1960s. Movies are made again. Second, there is a theme in which the hero is a lost child (*The Kid* or *Big*) and frequently an adult who is returned to childhood for a sort of a second chance at it. In this fictive return, which is clearly the place of powerful moral imagination, the childhood is in the 1950s (even when the age of the present character would not allow a 1950s childhood). Often in these fantasies, again contra actual demographics, there is an immigrant grandparent, to whom the kid bonds. The child is seen as happy, free, and authentic; the adult is seen as sad, pathetic, even pathological, and as artificial, not "natural," and not free. Here, the link between the morality of childhood and the happy freedom of childhood is powerfully made. To be a good person, say these persistent cultural narratives, is to be a happy child.

Play as Liberation

Linked to the syntax of childhood linguistic styles is the notion that full human flourishing is achieved through various forms of playful exertion. Unlike exertion in the course of the work of adult life—building railroads or farming or chasing animals—exercise has two functions. First, it celebrates and continues recess as a part of daily life. Further, it reifies the idea that one might, if one exercises enough, avoid death or old age entirely. The media is full of images that promise, "This is the face of 60." This is to mean that sixty-year-olds should look young and fit, and that the proper activity for elderly people is vigorous playful activity, often specially designed games, as on cruise ships, and not, for example, contemplation, study, or writing.

The Flight from Intergenerational Responsibility

When the idea of a funded Social Security retirement was presented in the 1930s and then reified in the 1960s with Medicare funding, the argument was made that after sixty-five, one would be too infirm to earn a living. The idea was to support elderly people so that their adult children would not be unduly impoverished by their care. Early images of this include the notion that the grandparents in a family turn their attention in their retirement to the care and education of grandchildren, allowing adults to work, and in many cultures, both agrarian and urban, this is still largely the case.[3] However, in American culture, retirement is seen, advertised, and enacted as a kind of long play period instead of a time of wisdom, reflection, the passing of the meme, and the acquisition of the responsibility to provide for one's progeny. A popular bumper sticker in Florida's Sun Coast reads, "I am spending my children's inheritance." Entire communities of retired adults are founded not only on the premise that one would not want to live with one's own grandchildren but also that one would rather not see or hear any children whatsoever. Grandparents are urged to flee as far as possible from their families, and the economies of several states depend on this idea, that one flees the phase of adulthood that is devoted to the tasks of attention to the next generation and goes golfing instead. And in these places, as in the larger culture, the expectation of happiness as constant as the Arizona sunshine is promised. Antidepressants are commonly prescribed, since, in the words of one gerontologist, "the feelings of sadness that are often a part of aging just don't have to be there anymore."[4]

In such a cultural shift, the idea of intergenerational responsibility becomes a rare choice, hardly seen as an integral part of adult life and the necessary obligations of such life in a society of responsible adults. People who make moral choices that involve avoiding or fleeing from the commitments of adult life, such as marriage, children, grandchildren, care of the elderly, and care of family or infirm friends, often make a moral argument like that of a teenager: that true selfhood is expressed by taking the least responsible course. Authenticity is linked to the ability to carry the minimal load—to "pack light" and to be without the "baggage" or burden of family, promises, or even memory. Looking ahead, reinventing the self as a younger, freer self-as-child is seen as the happier, healthier choice; one is admonished to abandon difficult persons, to avoid their need for you, lest one be a codependent. Hence the entire premise of adulthood—that one can be counted

LAURIE ZOLOTH

on in sickness and in health—is undercut by the idea that one can leave those entanglements and communities that require too much of oneself. In fact the idea, expressed in Emmanuel Levinas, that one gives the very skin of the self to the other, and one carries the other's life and even unfilled responsibilities, is seen as a kind of pathology, for which, of course, we have a medication: Prozac.

Care of the Dying in Philosophy

It is not only retirement that is reconfigured as a kind of flight, or dependency relationships that are seen as deniable. It is the entire embodied experience of any aging at all that is at stake. Consider the cell-by-cell delicacy of the hair turning gray, the way the hair of the body slowly turns into the pure silver light of the aging self. Once seen as the grace of wisdom manifested and inscribed on the body,[5] the first gray hair is routinely seen as a form of dreadful and disgraceful disfigurement.

Hair is routinely dyed in both men and women. Unlike in the 1950s, the effect is not to transform the self from dowdy to fabulous—since it is a rare person who actually goes platinum blond. Hair is dyed to deny the body itself. Here we have the widespread phenomenon of intellectuals, academics, and public leaders simply pretending that they do not have the gray hair that is a normal concomitant of adulthood, and they can choose to return to the color they had, which is to say pretend that they are the self they were, at, say, age seventeen.

What makes this particularly disturbing is that many who dye their hair are specialists in the kind of philosophy (bioethics) or theology or psychology that claims expertise in care of the dying. The color of choice is a sedate brown, often a henna dye, so one can think of this as a health store, "natural" sort of affair. Of course, even as the philosopher or geriatric specialist or theologian carefully reads the paper describing the merits of aging or the proper way to regard the dying process, she or he has inscribed her or his very body to enact the sentence, "But not me! I am not an old person! I am still in the body of the grad student!"

In thinking in this way, I want to turn our attention to the power of the signs that each of us are for one another. What makes this small gesture of pretend so powerful is precisely that it is so widespread, so common, and so understandable. Such a gesture was once only seen in film stars,[6] whereby the aging male star, via hair dye and makeup and by dating young women, could "play" young men. But such a "play" of the part of the happy ingenue is now available to all. One stands in front of the mirror, and one cannot come to terms with the face that one cannot cancel. It bears the truth of finality, of fragility; it is the mask of death, and one flees—one flees dying with dying, as in the old, first children's game of hide and seek. If you cover your face, you are invisible to the foe.

So, too, faith traditions—seen in eras past as the carriers of the tradition; the places of long, slow apprenticeship; the institutions that valued the wisdom of patriarchs and matriarchs and that cared for old texts and adult experiences—have in many cases felt the need to attract followers from the baby boomer generation with an elaborate insistence on play. In this, all mention of the sacred canopy of religion in the face of death[7] or of the centrality of the Christian narrative of death and resurrection[8] or of the crisis of liberation and commandment of Judaism[9] is avoided. In many faith traditions, all attempts at discipline, dues regulation, timeliness, study, and so forth have been abandoned, with attendant efforts to prove the "fun" and "unstructured" or "free" nature of the experience, precisely as if one were advertising a day care center.[10] Even in religious events, actual children may not be provided for carefully, since it is the adults who are instructed to act like children themselves, to "be cool."[11] One is urged with guitars and junk food to be joyful, to skip the Latin, or to avoid what might be the actual implications of a religious life, meaning to be bound, *ligiea*, to one another or to pray as if it were a matter of life and death.

PART 2: THE REALITY OF ILLNESS IN A CULTURE OF HAPPINESS

There is on a trail I know a certain kind of stone. In it, you can see the dark veins of the coal—dead possibilities, old stories of plants gone to death and weight and opacity. The stone breaks along these veins; the slightest whack and it fractures. I have a friend like that, I think, as I turn the stone in my hand, with clinical depression so profound that it has cut across his life in dark fault lines. I do not know all the reasons why this is so. Perhaps he is like the stone, and whatever has happened in the living story of his family, under the weight of crushing years, lives in him; or it may be genetic. One reads of long-acting viruses or of birth injuries—depression is a complex illness.[12]

LAURIE ZOLOTH

Knowing this reality interrupts the social criticism that I just undertook in the first pages of this essay, and it presents a serious challenge to my own argument: surely one cannot deny that some depression is an illness for which medicine has finally found a cure?

What I do know about the reality of despair is that for my friend, and for the many who struggle with significant clinical depression, it takes up such residence in the body that who one is becomes primarily gestures of anger and sorrow, and that one cannot wash dishes or cut up tomatoes or drive a car without being furious at something in one's path, and that fury fills the room with anger. But when the medications work, for many it is precisely like the claims of the ads for selective serotonin reuptake inhibitors (SSRIS) in the *New England Journal* or the *Journal of the American Medical Association.* Transformed, they say, "I am myself again." It is like the self—the "real" self that one's friends recognize as their buddy—is over for a while for a visit from out of town, and the other guy, the irritable, miserable, jumpy one, is gone. When the SSRIS do not work well, the darkness begins, and this one has eerily left his or her self again. It is like knowing a fragile, insulin-dependent diabetic, one whose consciousness is in the grip of a narrow band of chemical reactions, and if out of the band faces mortal peril. One sees the mood take over the face and the posture, closing and shrinking the body. A colleague writes to me about his wife, how it was to come home with his baby son and find her unconscious in the bathroom or sobbing uncontrollably on the sofa and to carry her to the hospital—of how this happens over and over. At times he writes of her recoveries or of new treatments. Once, they wrote an article together describing her return to wellness. Then I meet him at a conference and he tells me about her relapse into despair, and this cycle goes on for years. When I tell people I am writing this article, for example, colleagues and friends are eager to tell me about their treatment, how the medication restored them "to themselves," or how they know someone on the drugs and how it works for them.

Every article on Prozac has this caveat, and this article is no different: for the person with serious clinical depression, antidepressant medications are a lifesaving medical intervention. My friends literally owe their lives to them. As everyone who writes of SSRIS knows, the world that Prozac has made also contains stories like these, of recovery or at least of some meaningful moments of respite from a catastrophic world collapsed. In point of fact, I have come to believe that this condition is both helped by antidepressants and in a way potentiated by the culture that is shaped by/is shaping their use. Sorrow is

Care of the Dying in America   111

now against a ground of increasing expectations of cheerfulness and youthful energy, in which illness pulls against powerful social forces as a background. Unlike other eras, in which the tubercular, the fragile, or the sensitive person had a cultural location as a member of the genre of serious, introspective, analytic public intellectualism, the model of the discourse is one of unrelenting upbeatness.

Adult life is, in truth, a series of losses: not only does the hair turn silver, like metal beaten over and over, but it is the heart that is beaten that way. To be a parent is to see a child first grow from the tininess of one's hand into a person who will walk away from you into their own life, to learn to steadily bicycle down the street, growing smaller, receding into the distance of the road ahead. To live as an adult is to lose some serious battles with powers and authorities greater than you, to become decentered, to have to feel miserable, and to have to get up the next day, trying the task again. To live as an adult in a community of others is to see the failures of others and to take up their failures, their responsibilities, as one's own.

Being a being in time and across time means, like all living organisms, dying into the next phase, but slowly, and with consciousness of each loss. The heaviness of grief, the sickness at the center of the chest—this is not a new sort of illness. This is the existence and essence of beings in time, living alert to the one breathing next to you, wary of his danger and necessarily entrusted with his life. The taking on of the "yoke of the kingdom of Heaven" in classic Jewish thought is the taking on of the commanded life. It is a life of obligation, an agonistic and tempted journey, and the experience of the journey is surely not one of unremitting sorrow but is not one of simple happiness either.

The many who have written of this make a serious claim for their illness and its treatment. In a richly documented book on depression, Andrew Solomon not only describes his disease and recovery but notes the widespread occurrence of clinical depression: "Though it is a mistake to confuse numbers with truth, the numbers tell an alarming story. According to recent research, about 3 percent of Americans—some 19 million—suffer from chronic depression. . . . Depression as described in the DSM-IV is the leading cause of disability in the United States and abroad for persons over the age of five. . . . Depression claims more years than war, cancer, and AIDS put together."[13]

Such a statement derives its potency from the way that Solomon and his sources understand and perceive illness itself: "Other illnesses, from alcoholism to heart disease, mask depression when it causes them; if one takes that into consideration, depression may be the biggest killer on earth."[14] In other words, depression is essential, primal, and first cause of physical illness in this account. As Solomon notes as well, this disease understanding has led to dramatic new treatments. But even so, the medications are hardly addressing the problem:

> About 28 million Americans—one in every ten—are now on SSRIS . . . , and a substantial number are on other medications. . . . Twenty years ago, about 1.5 percent of the population had depression that required treatment, now it is 5 percent; and as many as 10 percent of all Americans now living can expect to have a major depressive episode during their life. About 50 percent will experience some symptoms of depression. Clinical problems have increased, treatments have increased vastly more. Diagnosis is up, but that does not explain the scale of the problem. Depression is increasing across the developed world. . . . Things are getting worse.[15]

Yet "things," especially in the developed world, are not getting worse. The usual measures for quality of life all show remarkable improvement. The economy has driven this, of course, and new technology, but other factors over the same twenty-year period might argue for an increased social optimism. Civic and civil freedoms have increased through serious discourse about the law and public policy: women, gays, the disabled community, and minorities have achieved many of the goals of the 1960s. Americans are not being drafted for a war in Vietnam, parklands are being restored, attention is newly given to the environment, public spaces are smoke free, and book clubs exist and are a growing phenomenon. Infant mortality is down, and so is teenage pregnancy. Why, and why now, is the phenomenon of despair—the despairing, anxious, and desperately, mortally ill body—so much a part of our culture?

PART 3: WALTER BENJAMIN, HANNAH ARENDT, AND GERSHOM SCHOLEM DISCUSS KAFKA

In this section of this essay, I explore the question of whether there is something to be learned about culture, self, depression, and response that might help us to answer the question I just raised. Here, I turn to a Europe that newly understands the world of Sigmund Freud and the inner world, especially the inner world of the German Jew, the subject of much of the analysis via which Freud created the discipline of psychotherapy. Despair is treatable, an illness with a cure, the "talking cure," and not a matter of sin. But the inner world itself is under siege. How do the idea of depression and the idea of its cure fare in this world? What can this narrative tell us about adults facing terror and the fear of death?

It is 1933 in the darkening hours of European Jewry; philosopher Walter Benjamin sends a letter to his friend Gershom Scholem, a historian. They discuss the work of their friend, the young philosopher Hannah Arendt. She is writing a manuscript about assimilation; she is traveling to Jerusalem with a boatload of orphans. Scholem has known since age fourteen that he is a Zionist, and after attending the university with Benjamin, he leaves for a life in Palestine, yearning for "an Israel." Like Benjamin, who must flee Germany to exile and desperate danger in occupied France, Scholem's life is lived in a most dangerous place, where being a Jew, one's very body, merely living in that particular self, is a dangerous act. There are riots against Jews in both places, and in both Europe and Palestine, friends disappear, cannot be rescued, and are killed. Benjamin's brother, and Scholem's as well, already is in a Nazi prison from which he will never escape.

Still, there are places that are free as yet. They write of the possibility of travel, and they write to each other about America, where Scholem is invited to lecture, and about the "comfortable and droll existence" there,[16] in the midst of a world careering toward the Shoah:

> It's a most attractive country, where life is easy if only you have sufficient means at your disposal. . . . The detachedness people have regarding what is happening to them is still very much unstrained which is great as far as their own affairs are concerned, but drives you mad where European or global affairs are concerned. On the whole, not a soul is interested in what is happening outside of his corner of the globe. . . . I would be happy to spend a whole year there sometime, but I imagine it would be unbearable in the long run.[17]

America was a Disneyland for them; yet it was unbearable to live there, since there were adult things to do—write philosophy and make meaningful choices, trying to save, first, literature and culture and, finally, a people from erasure. To flee from that task would be "unbearable." Living in their adult world was to live with the sense of death everywhere. And yet both men were relatively young, in their forties, as they wrote to each other; they lived out an entire, adult, elegant, and curious literary life against this sense—not in denial of death, but in light of it. They argue about the nature of truth and whether it is possible, or whether there exists "only the possibility of its transmission through centuries of interpretation."[18] They debate the nature of *galut* (exile) and the "inner nihilism of Judaism itself," in which "all that befalls the world is only an expression of this primal and fundamental galut. All existence, including God, subsists in galut." In this, Scholem is speaking out of his sense that the solution to catastrophe was a radical return—to the core of Judaism, to the land of Israel, to secret and difficult, lost Hebrew texts.[19] For Benjamin, all aspects of human existence, even and including the very language, the writing that will become all that he has against the terror of his existence, are fallen from an Adamic state. Language, too, is in exile, confounded by ambiguity and distanced by its use as a means to declare war, to describe "things," as opposed to its real task as "the human expression of the inexpressible." They are living in a world that has abandoned them: "I have no homeland, no fatherland, no friends anymore, everything that once clung to me has abandoned me to assume new bonds."[20]

What are we to do? they ask in the letters, and they have strategies for the adult life of loss and death. Scholem will, in this period, write his magisterial book on Jewish messianism—reflecting on the idea that a messianic hopefulness is only possible if one is aware of the totality of catastrophe. It is not happiness that is pursued, and certainly not childhood, not a return to their past.

Benjamin will write of the meaning in ordinary life, beginning work on his Arcades Project, the manuscript he will carry with him to his death. Benjamin writes to philosopher Theodor Adorno that "the attempt to retain the image of history in the most inconspicuous concerns of existence" might be "the actual, if not the only reason, not to abandon courage in the struggle for existence." It is the ordinal life, of friendship, of objects of daily use, and of narratives, that provides a source for this courage. It is difficult to write and to live in danger, money is scarce, and the exile deepens; yet they continue: "The absolute impossibility of having anything at all to draw on threatens a person's inner equilibrium in the long run." They discuss the struggle and the meaning of returning to settle in Jerusalem, and the project that their friend, the young philosopher Hannah Arendt, undertakes, to direct the rescue of endangered Jewish children by sending them to safety in Jerusalem—an illusive safety, as some will die in Arab attacks. But she is desperate, seeing the necessity of the temporal act of parental responsibility; at least some may survive, and in this she assumes the role of parent to these children. The quest for sanity is in figuring out how to be older, wiser, wise beyond one's years, taking care and taking responsibility for the political and against the social. Scholem cannot rescue Benjamin, can barely see Arendt, and fears that "murder and manslaughter are inevitable" in the riots in Jerusalem—"the future of Judaism is totally cloaked in darkness."[21] The way out of despair, they write, seriously and soberly, is only through courage. They do not expect happiness. They are looking, rather, for truth.

In the midst of the accounts of war, riot, and the collapse of European Jewry and the world they have shared, the three scholars—Scholem, Arendt, and Benjamin—write to one another of Franz Kafka, the Jew at the end of the German world whose ill body is a metaphor for the condition of the Jew, whose theme is transformation and disguise, the metamorphosis that is a kind of dying. Kafka represents a way to speak of the problem they face without personal despair overtaking them. *Is there a possibility of truth in the world?*

Benjamin writes,

> It is (this) consistency of truth that has been lost. Kafka was far from being the first to face this situation. Many had accommodated themselves to it, clinging to truth or what ever they happened to regard as such, and with a more or less heavy heart, had renounced transmissibility. Kafka's real genius was that he tried something entirely new: he sacrificed truth for the sake of clinging to transmissibility, to its aggadic [narrative] element. . . . But that is their misery and their beauty, that they had to be more than parables. They do not modest lie at the feet of doctrine as aggadah lies at the feet of halachah [Law]. When they have crouched down, they unexpectedly raise a mighty paw against it. This is why in the case of Kafka, we can no longer speak of wisdom. Only the products of its decay remain. There are two: One is the rumor about true things . . . ; the other is . . . folly. This much Kafka was absolutely sure of: First, that someone must be a fool if he is to help, and that only a fool's help is real help. The only uncertain thing is: Can such help still do a human being any good? . . . Thus as Kafka puts it, there is an infinite amount of hope, but not for us.[22]

Kafka's "serenity" emerges from his "certainty in his sense of failure."[23] But Kafka is important to our understanding of the situation they face, not only because of his narratives about the collapse of the truth claims of modernity but because of his choice of discourse. Kafka defines the state of existential despair not as "unhappiness" but as "illness"—the "discourse of the tubercular," a subject that he takes up as a central metaphor of his work long before he himself is diagnosed with the tuberculosis that will take his life in 1925, as Sander Gilman reminds us.[24] Kafka inhabits the tubercular, ill, "nervous" body: his chest is heavy, tight with grief, and it is difficult to breath without panic: "What did Franz Kafka see when he looked in the mirror? Or what did he imagine he saw?" Gilman notes Kafka's sense of his body as failed: "It is certain that a major obstacle to my progress is my physical condition. Nothing can be accomplished with such a body. . . . Everything is pulled about throughout the length of my body. What could it accomplish then, when it perhaps wouldn't have enough strength for what I want to achieve . . . ?"[25] The dis-ease of the time is not depression, but nervous unease. Gilman understands that this fin de siècle sense of the Jewish body as illness personified haunts the medical writings of the period. There is confusion in these texts about the actual spread of the disease, tuberculosis, and the psychological interplay of the symptomology with the essential state of the Jew, a confusion that will deepen into the idea that the German body politic needs to be cleansed of the Jewish body itself.[26] Writing of the Jew as diseased, Anatole Leroy-Beaulieu notes, "The Jew is particularly liable to this disease of our age, neurosis. . . . The Jew is the most nervous, and, in so far, the most modern of men. He is, by the very nature of his disease, the forerunner as it were, of his contemporaries, preceding them on the perilous path upon which society is urged by the excesses of its intellectual and emotional life, and by the increasing spur of competition."[27] Indeed, Kafka's first signs of tuberculosis are diagnosed as "nervousness," which in our time would be, of course, depression, and would line him right up for a series of SSRIs. If in Germany in the 1920s and 1930s the obsession was with difference, the urge to escape inscribed by Kafka as mutability or fantasy or the yearning for a "compact" powerful body, by the 1940s such doors had closed. There was no metamorphosis from the penal colonies that were the "cure" for the Jew's disease.

The intricate discussion proceeds between them: What is truth and what is justified? What is the warrant for any serenity? But serenity and hope cannot be found in the landscape of the past.

A Violent Courage of Life

Looking back on these letters, we, who live in the American social world that is "droll" and increasingly so, see how utterly understandable it is that these quixotic Europeans could not imagine enduring the oblivious, self-directed concerns of the happy Americans, for any period of time. The pursuit of happiness, as Carl Elliott reminds us, can tend to turn on oneself, and in this I am reminded of Kafka's metaphoric knife—turning to cut from the front, then from the back. The philosophers struggle to find the authentic life, of resistance and of creativity, even in terrible sorrow. They resist until the very end. Walter Benjamin walks over the Pyrenees, nearly out, carrying his manuscript, but arrives late, and hours before, the border had been closed. He is to be sent back to what he knows is certain torture and certain death in a concentration camp, and trapped, he kills himself. It is a question heard everywhere in 1942—it is, of course, the great question of all clinical depression as well. Arendt, in the camp at Gurs writes, "I heard only once about suicide, and that was the suggestion of a collective action, apparently a kind of protest in order to vex the French. When some of us suggested that we had been shipped there pour crever [to be done in], in any case, the general mood turned suddenly into a violent courage of life."[28] The prisoners understood that the "whole accident" of what had befallen them (her phrase) was not "personal and individual," and so the act of suicidal despair was an "asocial" and fundamentally "unconcerned" one. To be in the world, to "love the world," in her phrase, or to come as a lover into the world, as in the images of the Talmudic discourse, is to see one's despair as fundamentally social, requiring relationality and solidarity to alter. It is to be fundamentally concerned, fundamentally responsible.

Arendt, hearing of Walter Benjamin's death, writes about the placement of the self in time, to be a witness and a bearer of time, meaning a constancy of conscience and nowness, alert to the "small archaic" yet sustaining voices of the past and aware of the necessity of one's journey into the thenness of the future. Placement of the self into time in this way is not only a designation of courage; it is an ethical gesture as well. It is a poem of loss, of course, for her friend "W. B." and a poem about one's own moral location in the open face of loss. And it is a record, of course, of what can be seen as what she understands and what will turn out to be truthful at the end, that even this most lost one was a person we can claim as ours, to whom we are responsible as fellows, another in our crowded time and proximity. It is a way to see a way out of sorrow—the only way, finally—to be social, possible, difficult:

W. B.

Dusk will come again sometime.
Night will come down from the stars.

We will rest our outstretched arms
In the nearness, in the distances.

Out of the darkness sound softly
small archaic melodies. Listening,
let us wean ourselves away,
let us at last break ranks.

Distant voices, sadness nearby.
These are the voices and these are the dead
whom we have sent as messengers
ahead, to lead us into slumber.[29]

Heimatlos

Hannah Arendt narrowly escapes from the war and becomes a leading American philosopher, aging into her beautiful graying body and
writing always of the grief and the trials and the temptations toward
insignificance in the human condition. Her complex grief and yearning for the lost world of Europe is rooted in the complexity of the exilic
condition itself. There is no going back to childhood. In another poem
written in 1946, after the war, she writes of *heimatlos*, homelessness,
and of despair and its discontents:

Sorrow is like a light that gleams in the heart
Darkness is a glow that searches our night
We need strike only the small, mournful flame
To find our way home, like shadows, through the
    long, broad night.
The woods, the city, the street, the tree are
    luminous.
Lucky is he who has no home; he sees it still
    in his dreams.[30]

Philosophy, in the sense that these writers mean it, is a recognition that the self lives against temporality, in that it is both aware of
the consciousness of the self and the ironic "failure" of the self to be
the imagined self-in-culture. At its best, notes Arendt, sorrow is not
denied, but "gleams in the heart." For Benjamin, despair is not an unfamiliar part of the essential stance of the human person who is aware
of the desert of modernity. It will only be the transformative power of
words, imagination, a choice to "safeguard what we hold in common"
in the fastness of friendship. In his last letter to Scholem, Benjamin

notes the horror of his situation but looks forward to seeing his friend in the future and "falling" into each other's arms, asking him to attend to "the markers in the desert landscape of the present that cannot be overlooked by old Bedouins like us."[31] That will be offered as the resistance to the understanding of the desperate situation of the self in modernity.

PART 4: RUMORS OF TRUE THINGS:
INCORPORATION AND COMMUNAL LOSS

Hence, we can place the story of these moments in history in which young men and women were forced to and did act with serious intent and did not deny the gravity of their situation, against the culture we all face but did deny the temptation to act as a child, and a frivolous one at that. But it was not only toward philosophy that the Jewish intellectuals named here turned; it was also to a complex apprehension of their engagement with their Judaism itself. It is my contention that such a turn is a reasonable one. In this final conversation of this essay, I argue for a classic text and practice that normalizes despair from within a particular theological tradition. Benjamin claims that passing on the truthful rumor is why theology is important, the rumor of what cannot, finally, be proved, but what must be only believed. Hence, following Benjamin, Scholem, and Arendt, where does one turn for the sources for the "violent courage"? Classically, the sources of Jewish thought can teach much about the problem of exile, and of the tragic necessity of living on after the worst has happened. I want to claim that one can find the consolation and the witness to the exilic state in which we live if one turns from our America of "comfortable and droll existence" to a thoughtful consideration of one's actual situation of exile from the possible, to the understanding that of course one must live in exile, having left the country of childhood behind. To be an adult is to know this, and to know how hard the thing is, and how elusive serenity is. Literature is one way to tell of how hard and sad it can be.

Of course it is sad: to live in the face of death always would take courage, and it is an overwhelming task to face this alone, without community, without actual faith, without citizenship, without friendship, and without intergenerational families at your side. It is no wonder that one wants to be a child with a Mommy who is nearby, with toys at your feet, rather than be a graying lady with a job in the morning, many children to feed, a set of forms to complete, and the Grand Inquisitor coming at noon who will be wearing a grin and a "Hi, Call Me Nancy" badge. It is no wonder that in the 1950s one wanted a drink and a box of chocolate, and in the 2000s one yearns for Prozac.

Reasoning from a Rumor of Truth-Life in Exile

But there are rumors of truth in the aggadic narratives of the Talmud, and I know them; so I will at least pass these along. It is the understanding that Arendt articulates, that tragedy is never utterly personal, which is at the core of the account of the Jewish theological stance. One is not only a being in time, held and bound to and by time, held and bound to and by history; one is also a being in society, in "the social" as well as the polis and the family.

In the Jewish calendar there is an annual holiday of grief, the ninth day of the Jewish month of Av (Tisha b'Av). On this day, one is supposed to, well, be sad, excessively, formally so. It is an immersion in "the greatest sorrow imaginable." One sits on the ground, one is prohibited from wearing leather shoes, one fasts, one takes on the affect of formal mourning rituals, and the entire community reads the Book of Lamentations, Eichah, by candlelight in a darkened synagogue. As one reads Eichah on this day, one laments a collection of griefs: the biblical event in which the spies gave a negative report of the land of Israel, thus beginning the first exilic forty years of wandering after the Exodus from Egypt; the destruction of the First Temple (586 B.C.E.) and the Second Temple (70 C.E.); the defeat of the Bar Kochba rebellion and the fall of Beitar; the ploughing of Jerusalem (135); the expulsion of the Jews from England (1290); the Spanish Inquisition (1492); and the beginning of the selections in the Warsaw Ghetto.[32] All of these events, of course, are the "markers set up in the desert of exile"—the people, in this account are "Bedouins" in space and in time. It is an oddly efficient concept (this gathering of all the worst events into one day) and an odd enactment (acting just as if the death had really just happened that day). The day ends with rituals to suggest that only after deepest despair is messianic hope possible, and in an odd practice, one prepares one's home by sweeping the floor in anticipation of the Messiah, and the day ends with this little ordinary hopeful sign.

Just six days later, there is another holiday, Tu b'Av, and this day, the Talmud suggests in an ironic linguistic solution to despair, is a time of "the greatest joy imaginable." Women exchange white dresses and, wearing one another's clothes, in a gesture of radical, embodied social solidarity, come out to dance in the vineyards and meet young men and pair off into marriage. But even as this is said in the Talmudic description, it is unsaid with an objection from another rabbinic authority: What is so great about this random day that it might serve as some response to the momentous grief we just were commanded to enact? How does ritual serve against memory of the great abandonment that Benjamin understands, at least, as utter aloneness, not just of the self, but of the people? Here is the text in which they debate the problem of how one is supposed to act on this second day:

> Mishnah: R. Simeon b. Gamliel said: There never were in Israel greater days of joy than the fifteenth of Av and the Day of Atonement (Yom Kippur). On these days, the daughters of Israel used to walk out in white garments which they borrowed in order not to put to shame any one who had none . . . exclaiming at the same time, young man, lift up thine eyes and see what thou choosest for thyself. Do not set thine eyes on beauty, but set thine eyes on (good) family. Grace is deceitful and beauty is vain; but a woman that fears the Lord, she shall be praised. . . . Give her the fruit of her hands; and let her works praise her in the Gates.

> Gemora: I can understand the Day of Atonement, because it is a day of forgiveness and pardon and on it the Second Tables of the Law were given, but what happened on the fifteenth of Av? [33]

I am turning to this text in my final discussion about depression, despair, and death precisely because it is a complex text about resiliency—and intergenerational responsibility and, finally, the necessity of taking up the task of adult life in the face of terror, loss, and despair, surrounded by others, meaning the others of history and the others of your future in that one's task is to turn from the ritual reenactment of despair to the liturgical hint of marriage and dinner (the phrase "Give her the fruit of her hands" in the last sentence of the Mishnah being taken from the Book of Proverbs and said in praise of a wife at a traditional Shabbas meal). It is a text about fecundity and continuity and social community in the face of death, rather than flight and denial or superficial illusions of physical beauty, which itself repeats in the law. In reflecting on this text, Yair Silverman noted that what is "celebrated" in the Talmud are four equivocal events:[34] the ability to marry between the tribes of Israel and to reestablish the tribe of Benjamin after all the men of the tribe were killed by the rest of the tribes in the nation to punish them for an act of horror; the end of the deaths of the first generation of the slaves exiled into the desert; the lifting of the Roman decree that the bodies of the rebels of Bar Kochba would have to rot in the open; and the anniversary of the removal of guards on the road to Jerusalem, set up by a misguided king. Hardly joyful, these events, argues Silverman, are precisely minimalist in nature and represent the ability to find something, even at the last, to celebrate, to turn from despair into a new chance. The events are the social equivalent of the little act of sweeping the floor, an Arcades Project sort of act, one that Benjamin himself might have appreciated, this holiness at the core of ordinary life.

The year turns on this day, typically at the end of summer, when, subtly, the sun's power is lessened—a good thing in a desert land—and the sense of possibility that rain will come, and harvest can be made, is faintly, altogether faintly, reasserted. It is the Jewish contention that God-in-Exile may not remove despair or cheer us all up but is, in the sense that Scholem, Benjamin, and Arendt understood, in witness to us, in solidarity with us, in the Exile as well. What one has, then, is merely/totally presence—the answer to the question, Where are you? This is the central question of recognition that the biblical text has God first ask of Adam, then Noah, and then, finally, Abram before it is correctly answered: I am right here! And in a sense, this is the essential question of depression: Where is everyone, where truth or even its rumors, where goodness, where the adults to care for me, where God? Unlike Adam, who hides, or Noah, who is silent before the question, the correct response is to prepare for the next task, alert to the need.

In the liturgy of Tisha b'Av, the holy day of grief, the texts ask, Am I alone in this exile? Are we just careering toward deeper exile, not the Temple, not even the Land, not even Vilna? It is asked, this time, of God in the text, by the people lost in their despair, which can be seen, notes scholar Ellen LeVee, in a linguistic trick:[35] a transmutation of the Hebrew to form the word "how" by which the Book of Lamentations is known in Jewish tradition (both "how" and "where are you" are spelled aleph-yod-kawf-heh), and the answer is annually, liturgically, the same, *hineni* (I am right here). What is "right here" in exile is the Law and the practice, carried only in community. Alone, all would be lost in despair: hence, the necessity to sweep the house, to wear the clothes of your sister, to dance, to think about bodies and sexuality and babies and dinner again.

It is my contention that careful thinking about that idea is only a rumor, but it is a helpful one indeed, a small thing; and like a drug, it might only last for a while, and then one would have to think about it again.[36] It is this refusal to turn from the exilic moment or the terrible realization of the collapse of all hope that is what is required in adult life, and I would argue that it is probably only bearable if one has a coherent practice, narrative, faith, and task in a community of other exiles. It is the great temptation to deny the terror of this choice, to turn from the necessity to do work that is praiseworthy and bear fruit that is tangible, useful, and that needs to be shared, sold, bartered, or given. It is an absurdity to think that anything, any falsity, any gaiety that is based on the countenance or the look of youth, any possession, even one's own clothes, can cover the problem.

CONCLUSION

Can text or history save us? Do my three interrupting conversations— deliberately, they are not completed, calling for further talk—suggest a response to ways we might live in a world of Prozac, Zoloft, and all the others? Can such reflection allow a distinction between sorrow as illness and sorrow as a sort of perception?

The project of thinking through what faces us in light of a story, especially within the Jewish tradition of philosophy, is the model for Benjamin, Arendt, and Scholem, for Kafka, and for the rabbinic culture that turns textually and linguistically within an interpretive community. I would argue that for us, too, it has better odds than pretending to be a little girl or boy or wishing that the world were not really the way it is. Jewish texts, given the long years of exile, seem to be of particular use, but here, I am offering them as a central metaphor. Being the being in time locates us in history and in the future. Can text carry everything? That it once did, of course, is only a partial answer, and it is surely not my claim—the disease of despair is deadly and the losses too terrible. I like science and wish that whole project well. But for most of us, I think it is not Prozac that we need; I think it is another person who is willing to tell us stories, hear stories, and talk about them. By this I mean not only particular, personal stories (like swept floors on a summer evening), but Story, in the rabbinic sense. I think, however, that it is precisely that the world is not so small, after all, and hence, we will always need large things to sustain us: faith in the face of the boundless dark, the endless smallness of the self against it, the whole deal of history and memory, and the ability of hope. "Lucky is he who has no home; he sees it still in his dreams."[37]

LAURIE ZOLOTH

1. National Public Radio, "Morning Edition," January 2002.

2. This follows a more general literary trend, in which even in adult literature, the references are to the popular culture of childhood, rather than to the Western canon. Contrast "The Wasteland," or *Moby Dick*, for example, with contemporary novels.

3. In China, for example, grandparents are largely the source of the day care workforce.

4. Quoted at a Robert Wood Johnson seminar on end of life issues.

5. See Shakespeare's *King Lear*, for example.

6. Or famously and now so ironically, in President Ronald Reagan.

7. See Peter Berger, *The Sacred Canopy: Elements of a Sociological Theory of Religion* (Garden City, N.Y.: Doubleday, 1967).

8. See Stanley Hauerwas, *Dispatches from the Front: Theological Engagements with the Secular* (Durham, N.C.: Duke University Press, 1994).

9. See Emmanuel Levinas, "The Pact," in *The Levinas Reader*, ed. Seán Hand, trans. Sarah Richmond (Oxford: Blackwell, 1989), 221–26.

10. A sign advertises "a place for dis-organized religion" on a Chabad House, Pacific Coast Highway, July 2001.

11. Jonathan Shoresh, "Cool Jews," *Tikkun Magazine*, June 1999.

12. Peter D. Kramer, *Listening to Prozac* (New York: Viking, 1993).

13. Andrew Solomon, *The Noonday Demon: An Atlas of Depression* (New York: Scribner, 2001), 25.

14. Ibid.

15. Ibid., 26.

16. Gershom Scholem, ed., *The Correspondence of Walter Benjamin and Gershom Scholem, 1932–1940* (New York: Shocken Books, 1989), 170.

17. Ibid., 235.

18. Ibid., xiii.

19. Ibid.

20. Ibid., xxvi.

21. Ibid., 255.

22. Ibid., 225.

23. Ibid., 226.

24. Sander Gilman, *Franz Kafka, the Jewish Patient* (New York: Routledge, 1995).

25. Ibid., 63.

26. Ibid., 243. See also other works by Gilman on this point.

27. Ibid., 63, as cited by Gilman.

28. Elisabeth Young-Bruehl, *Hannah Arendt: For Love of the World* (New Haven: Yale University Press, 1982), 154.

29. Ibid., 163.

30. Ibid., 188. Note that the poem is a reflection on a line from German poet Rainer Maria Rilke—"lucky is he who has a home."

31. Scholem, *Correspondence*, 262. This is an except from Benjamin's last letter before his death.

32. Michael Strassfeld, *The Jewish Holidays: A Guide and Commentary* (New York: Harper and Row, 1985), 90.

33. Talmud Balvi, Ta'anit, 26b and 30b.

34. Yair Silverman in lecture and personal communication, August 9, 2001. Yair Silverman is making the point that the tension between the two holidays is meant to allow an intellectual and emotive project as one moves annually between them.

35. Ellen LeVee, in reflections on an earlier version of this essay, September 30, 2003.

36. Hence the need to pray three times a day in Jewish practice, five times in Islamic practice, begins to be clear.

37. Young-Bruehl, *Hannah Arendt*, 188.

Pursued by Happiness
and Beaten Senseless
Prozac and the American Dream

Let us start with cases. These come from an essay by psychotherapist Maureen O'Hara and Walter Truett Anderson. The names have been changed, but the patients, they tell us, are real.

(1) Jerry feels overwhelmed, anxious, fragmented, and confused. He disagrees with people he used to agree with and aligns himself with people he used to argue with. He questions his sense of reality and frequently asks himself what it all means. He has had all kinds of therapeutic and growth experiences: Gestalt, rebirthing, Jungian analysis, holotropic breathwork, bioenergetics, the Course in Miracles, twelve-step recovery groups, Zen meditation, and Ericksonian hypnosis. He has been to sweat lodges, to the Rajneesh ashram in Poona, and to the Wicca festival in Devon. He is in analysis again, this time with a self-psychologist. Although he is endlessly on the lookout for new ideas and experiences, he keeps saying he wishes he could simplify his life. He talks about buying land in Oregon. He loved *Dances with Wolves*.

(2) Alec is forty-two, single, and for most of his life has felt lonely and alienated. He has never cared much about politics, considers himself an agnostic, and has never found a hobby or interest he would want to pursue consistently. He says he does not think he really has a self at all. He has had two stints of psychotherapy; both ended inconclusively, leaving him still with chronic, low-grade depression. Nowadays he is feeling a little better about himself. He has started attending a local meeting of Adult Children of Alcoholics. People at the meetings seem to understand and validate his pain; he is making friends there and believes he "belongs" for the first time since he left the military. But he confesses to his therapist that

he feels "sort of squirrelly" about it because he is not an adult child of an alcoholic. He is faking the pathological label in order to be accepted by the community, and he is not too sure he really buys into their twelve-step ideology, either.

(3) Beverly comes into therapy torn between two lifestyles and two identities. In the California city where she goes to college, she is a radical feminist; on visits to her midwestern hometown, she is a nice, sweet, square conservative girl. The therapist asks her when she feels most like herself. She says, "When I'm on the airplane."[1]

Spiritual emptiness, the search for a sense of self, alienation in the midst of abundance: are there traits any more American than these? These are themes that characterize some of the most memorable American art of the middle and late twentieth century: from the poetry of T. S. Eliot to that of Sylvia Plath, in fiction from Nathanael West and J. D. Salinger through Saul Bellow and Don DeLillo, from the plays of Tennessee Williams to the documentary films of Ross McElwee, and from the songs of Woody Guthrie to those of the Talking Heads. If we are to believe Alexis de Tocqueville, this kind of spiritual restlessness has been with us since the early days of the republic. "In America I saw the freest and most enlightened men, placed in circumstances the happiest to be found in the world; yet it seemed to me as if a cloud habitually hung upon their brow, and I thought them serious and almost sad even in their pleasures."[2]

In the decade or so since the development of the selective serotonin reuptake inhibitors (SSRIS), many thoughtful (and some not so thoughtful) voices have urged caution, or at least a damper on our enthusiasm for the drugs, most notably in the debate prompted by Peter Kramer's splendid book, *Listening to Prozac*. Scholars have worried that Prozac treats the self rather than proper diseases, that it alters personality, that it feeds dangerously into the American obsession with competition and worldly success, and that it offers a mechanistic cure for problems of the spirit, just as Walker Percy predicted in his novel *Love in the Ruins*, where psychiatrist Tom More treats existential ailments with his Ontological Lapsometer. But in the years since I first read Kramer's book, I have begun to suspect that the problem may go deeper than Prozac—that the problem is not merely Prozac but the stance of psychiatry itself and the reason psychiatry has such a hard time saying anything helpful about these spiritual ills. Ludwig Wittgenstein once wrote, "The sickness of a time is cured by an alteration

CARL ELLIOTT

in the mode of life of human beings, and it was possible for the sickness of philosophical problems to get cured only through a changed mode of thought and of life, not through a medicine invented by an individual."[3] He was talking about philosophy, not psychopharmacology, but the point is apt either way. At least part of the nagging worry about Prozac and its ilk is that for all the good they do, the ills that they treat are part and parcel of the lonely, forgetful, and often unbearably sad place where we live.

I am slightly reluctant to use the term "alienation," coming as it does with baggage that I do not necessarily want to take with me, but so be it; here, I think, it can serve a useful purpose. Alienation seems to describe at least some of the symptoms that bring people to the attention of a psychiatrist. How many patients this is, and whether Prozac actually cures them, remains to be seen. It may be very small in comparison with, say, the number who use Prozac for depression. But I take it from my psychiatric colleagues, from the case histories in Kramer's book and others, and from my many friends and acquaintances who have used the drug, that whether it affects alienation is at least an open question.

Alienation, it seems to me, differs from most of the descriptors that psychiatry ordinarily uses for psychiatric patients—descriptors like anxiety, obsessiveness, and even unhappiness. These descriptors describe internal psychic states. They are about (to use a slightly misleading metaphor) what is in my own head. Relationships with things outside myself can affect my happiness or unhappiness or, for that matter, my depression or my anxiety or my obsessions; if I am in a miserable job or if my relationship with my wife is on the rocks or even if (as we say down South) I am not right with God, I might be more unhappy or more anxious or depressed. But the concepts themselves are by and large measures of my internal psychic well-being.

This makes them different from alienation. Alienation generally describes an incongruity between the self and external structures of meaning—a lack of fit between the way you are and the way you are expected to be, say, or a mismatch between the way you are living a life and the structures of meaning that tell you how to live a life. Alienated people are alienated from something—their families, their cultures, their jobs, or their Gods. This is not a purely internal matter; it is not just in the alienated person's head. It is about a mismatch between a person and something outside him- or herself. This, I think, is why it makes some sense (although one could contest this) to say that a person should be alienated—that given his or her circumstances, alienation is the proper response. Some external circumstances call for alienation.

Alienation comes in many varieties, or so I think, many of which blur into one another. For the sake of simplicity, I will mention three, with the caveat that these divisions are artificial and overlapping. The first is a kind of personal alienation, a sense that you do not conform with social expectations of someone in your particular circumstances. It might be that your character does not quite fit into place as it should, so that you feel ill at ease among the other Princeton men or Milwaukee Rotarians or suburban high school cheerleaders. It may be that you feel alienated from the social role you are expected to occupy. You are not cut out to be a Washington political wife or a Virginia gentleman or the inheritor of the family hardware business. Or perhaps the direction in which your life is moving simply does not mesh with the way it is expected to move, like a New Hampshire housewife who at age fifty says this is not the life for me, divorces her husband, sells the house, and goes off to Swaziland with the Peace Corps. For North Americans, these may be the most familiar kinds of alienation. They seem to be characteristic of times when a person's identity is questioned or under reevaluation, such as when we are in our early twenties and are expected to decide what to do with our lives: What should I do for a living? Where should I live? Should I marry? If so, whom? Or in mid-life, when we look back on the decisions we have made and how they have turned out: Why did I marry him? Why didn't we have children? How in God's name did I wind up in accounting?

A second type of alienation that comes to mind, related to the first, is cultural alienation. This often involves the sense that a particular form of life is changing beneath your feet, and that you no longer have the equipment to manage in the new way. This kind of alienation seems to be a motivating force behind a lot of social criticism. You step outside your own socialization (or you are pushed) and look at your own culture from a standpoint of detachment. Perhaps the most extreme example of this kind of alienation would be characteristic of colonized and displaced peoples: Native Americans whose traditional ways of life have been erased, Hmong refugees marooned in Minnesota, or Pacific Islanders colonized by the U.S. military, so that instead of fishing and harvesting tropical fruit they subsist on a diet of imported canned foods. I take it that this is also part of what Cornel West is getting at when, writing of the disappearance of traditional African American social institutions, he states that "the major enemy of black survival in America is neither oppression nor exploitation but rather the nihilistic threat—that is, loss of hope and absence of meaning."[4]

Walker Percy hints at this sort of alienation in *The Last Gentleman*, which takes place at a time when the old South of honor and agrarian living and racial inequality is fading away and is being replaced by a new, Republican, Christian South of golf clubs and subdivisions and Old Confederacy Used Car lots. For Will Barrett, Percy's protagonist, the result is disorientation, a sense of not quite knowing how he fits into this new culture and what he is supposed to be doing there. In Barrett's family, Percy writes, "The great-grandfather knew what was what and said so and acted accordingly and did not care what anyone thought." But over the generations Barrett's family lost its knack for action and no longer knew just what was what. Barrett's father said he did not care what other people thought, but he cared. He wanted to act honorably and to be thought well of by others. "So living for him was a strain. He became ironical. For him it was not a small thing to walk down the street on an ordinary September morning. In the end he was killed by his own irony and sadness and by the strain of living out an ordinary day in a perfect dance of honor."[5]

But cultural alienation need not involve cultural change. In fact, perhaps the most recognizable symbols of American alienation are houses in the suburbs, which are seen as alienating precisely because of their static, anonymous conformity. In Richard Ford's novel *Independence Day*, the realtor Frank Bascombe says that buying a house comes with great anxiety because of that "cold, unwelcome, built-in-America realization that we're just like the other schmo, wishing his wishes, lusting his stunted lusts, quaking over his idiot frights and fantasies, all of us popped out of the same unchinkable mold."[6] In a society that values uniqueness and individuality, that says a fulfilled life is one in which you look inside yourself and discover your own particular values and talents, and that valorizes the rule-breaking, anti-establishment, boundary-transgressing antihero, there is something terrifying about looking deep inside and discovering that you are no different from the guy next door, that your life is just an average life, and that your story is so ordinary that it is not even worth telling. Anything that reminds you of this fact—anything that betrays the illusion that you are really, deep down, quite an extraordinarily unique individual—is going to cut very close to the bone indeed. It is enough to make you think about an antidepressant.

Which leads to a third variety of alienation, one that I will call (with some trepidation) existential alienation. This kind of alienation involves questioning the very terms on which a life is built. By virtue of when, where, and to whom we are born, we inherit a sense of what it is possible to do with a human life, what kinds of lives are honorable or pointless or meaningful. To be a southerner, a Jew, a Quebecoise, or an Irishman is to be born into a certain way of seeing and being in the world. This is part of what makes us who we are. But what happens to us, to our sense of who we are, when we come to believe that the values we have are really nothing more than the values we have—not God's will or the inevitable consequence of history or the product of enlightened reason? Calling into question your own form of life involves calling into question your own values, the very stuff out of which you are built. This is not just realizing that your own particular castle is constructed on thin air. It is realizing you are built out of air yourself. It is radically disorienting: the ultimate, dizzying high-wire act, like Wile E. Coyote after he runs off a cliff and does just fine until he glances down and realizes where he is standing.

Many of the case histories surrounding Prozac, like those at the start of this essay, gesture at this kind of alienation—the sense that not only do you not know what to do with your life, but you do not know what could possibly tell you what to do. The structures that might have given life its sense and meaning are now contested or in question. The result is not just the feeling that you are ill suited for your own particular form of life or that your form of life is fading away; rather, it is a calling into question of the foundations of any form of life. Why this job, this church, this country, this house? Why this particular way of going on when I get up in the morning? Why *any* particular way? The result of these kinds of questions can be the sense that no form of life can have the kind of justification that you feel you need. It is a sense that there is no rhyme and reason to your form of life other than the exigencies of biology and history, that the big picture is really nothing more than a big picture.

Erik Parens has suggested to me that the account I have given here does not do justice to every sort of alienation, at least as many philosophers have understood it, and that the most important sorts of alienation may arise not from anything external to the self but from features intrinsic to human life. Jean-Jacques Rousseau, for example, thought that we are alienated from our sexuality. Martin Heidegger thought that we become alienated from our essential nature as human beings when we do not face up to the fact that we will die. I think that Parens is for the most part right—and right in an especially insightful way—yet right only up to a point. There is no getting around the fact that we will all die, but alienation from our condition as mortal beings is never simply that; it is always a response to what our particular culture and age have made of our condition as mortal beings. To say, as Heidegger does, that living well requires anxiety in the face of not Being presupposes a framework of understanding that sees death as not Being (rather than, say, eternal life in the presence of God, or reincarnation, or any of the many other ways that people have thought of death). The fact that we modern westerners are alienated from our sexuality or our mortality does not mean that all human beings at all times have been or must be alienated from them. When we are alienated from features intrinsic to human life, we are never alienated solely from those features themselves but from the meaning that our culture and age have given them.

Alienation of any type might go together with depression, of course, but I suspect that the two do not necessarily go hand in hand. I used to talk about alienation and depression with Benjy Freedman, my friend and colleague in bioethics at McGill University who died in 1997. Benjy was a loyal friend, ferociously intelligent and darkly funny, a complicated man of deep moral integrity. Yet for the first couple of years I knew him, he would periodically descend into very black moods. He would come into his office, close the door, draw the blinds, and sit all day in semidarkness. Sometimes he was irritable and would get into bitter arguments even with his close friends. I do not think Benjy would disagree with me when I say that he was probably clinically depressed. In fact, he once told me as much himself. He had recently suffered the deaths of two close family members. But Benjy was also a deeply devout Orthodox Jew. He was as secure in his faith as anyone I have ever known. He loved his family and was at home in his community. When Benjy and I talked about existential questions like these, questions about alienation from your culture and not knowing who to be or what to do with your life, he would just shake his head and laugh. Once he told me he had no idea what I was talking about. These were questions with which he just could not connect. Which is not to say that he was not depressed or anxious or worried. He worried a lot about doing his duty, about whether he was doing sound intellectual work, and about whether he was doing a good job as a teacher. But for him, the broader structures of meaning within which these questions are located were uncontested. Unlike me: I was vaguely lost without (at least at that time) feeling particularly unhappy about it; an expatriate southerner with a German wife living in Quebec and thus expected to be somewhat dislocated; a Walker Percy reader and thus strangely at home in the community of the alienated; undepressed, perhaps, but unlike Benjy, utterly at sea when it came to these broader structures of meaning.

Yet what is left for those of us who are lost at sea? Apparently we have to make do with secular expertise, the professionals that Percy called the experts of the self. If we are alienated and impoverished and cannot figure out why, we turn to doctors, psychologists, advice columnists, self-help authors, personal trainers, alternative healers, philosophical counselors, or (let us admit it) ethicists, who will set us on the path to righteousness, personal fitness, and sound mental hygiene. Why am I unhappy? Because you (1) are fat, (2) are shy, (3) dress badly, (4) do not own a house/sport utility vehicle/cell phone, (5) do not like to cook or keep house, (6) have never been on television, (7) are unable to converse on a variety of topics, (8) have not settled on a meaningful career, (9) do not have stimulating hobbies or fulfilling recreational activities, or (10) have not yet found the five steps to uncovering your inner capacity for childlike joy and wonderment. Experts of the self create facilities such as the Geriatrics Rehabilitation Unit in Percy's *Love in the Ruins*, where old folks often grow inexplicably sad, despite the fact that their every need is met. "Though they may live in the pleasantest Senior Settlements where their every need is filled, every recreation provided, every sort of hobby encouraged, nevertheless many grow despondent in their happiness, sit slack and empty-eyed at shuffleboard and ceramic oven. Fishing poles fall from tanned and healthy hands. Golf clubs rust. Reader's Digests go unread. Many old folk pine away and even die from unknown causes like a voodoo curse."[7]

Here is the key to the problem psychiatry has with a notion like alienation. The measure of psychiatric success is internal psychic well-being. The aim of psychiatry is (among other things) to get rid of anxieties, obsessions, compulsions, phobias, and various other barriers to good social functioning. Within this framework, where the measure of success is psychic well-being through good social functioning, alienation is something to be eliminated. It is a psychiatric complaint. It is a barrier to psychic well-being. Whereas what I want to suggest is that maybe psychic well-being is not everything. Some lives are better than others, quite apart from the psychic well-being of the person who is leading them. I do not mean this in any ultimate, metaphysical sense. I am not arguing that God prefers some lives to others, or that some lives are better than others because they are more rational or well ordered. I just mean that the notion that some lives are better than others is part of the moral background to the way we live our lives. We all recognize that it is possible for a life to be a failure or a success, even if we are not always able to say exactly why. Percy himself puts it this way: "We all know perfectly well that the man who lives out his life as a consumer, a sexual partner, an 'other-directed' executive; who avoids boredom and anxiety by consuming tons of newsprint, miles of movie film, years of TV time; that such a man has somehow betrayed his destiny as a human being."[8]

Well, maybe. When I hear phrases like "destiny of a human being," I start to squirm. But I take Percy's larger point seriously: by ignoring such matters as how a person lives his life, by steadfastly refusing to pass judgment on whether the ideals he or she lives by are worthy or wasteful or honorable or demeaning, psychiatry can say nothing useful whatsoever about alienation. It places itself in the position of neutrality about the broader structures of meaning within which lives are lived, and from which they might be alienated. What could a psychiatrist say to the happy slave? What could he or she say to an alienated Sisyphus as he pushes the boulder up the mountain? That he would push the boulder more enthusiastically, more creatively, more insightfully, if he were on Prozac?

Already I can hear the protests. Do you want to deny Prozac to Sisyphus? Who are you to criticize him for taking it? Very well, then. Perhaps I spoke hastily. My purpose was not to level any moral criticism. Sisyphus may well be happier on an antidepressant. His psychic well-being will probably be improved. Certainly he is entitled to the drug, if his managed care organization will pay for it. I only wish to point out that his predicament is not simply a matter of his internal psychic well-being. Any strategy that ignores certain larger aspects of his situation is going to sound a little hollow.

Of course, taking account of the larger situation is not as simple as I make it sound. Neither pills nor psychotherapy can fix metaphysics. In his essay "Truth to Truth" Leszek Kolakowski writes about his idea for a spiritual "conversion agency," which would offer religious and ideological transformations for a fee. The most difficult conversions are the most expensive—say, to fundamentalist Islam or Albanian Communism. Lower fees are charged for less demanding, more comfortable belief systems, like Anglicanism or reform Judaism. The agency itself, however, needs to remain strictly neutral, in order to preserve the autonomy of patients. "Psychologists and other experts of indoctrination shall then be entrusted with the actual work, which will in no way violate the freedom of the individual. The agency itself must remain strictly neutral religiously and ideologically; it could be named Veritas, 'Truth,' or Certitudo, 'Certitude' (perhaps, 'Happy Certitude')."[9]

Kolakowski's satire gets the dilemma psychiatry has with these larger questions. Of course it makes sense to think that psychiatry should remain neutral on matters of religion and ideology. Show me a psychiatrist who sees the verities of Baptist theology as the solution to all his patients' problems, and I will show you a case of psychiatric malpractice. What Kolakowski is poking fun at, though, is the notion that spiritual affairs are matters upon which it is *possible* to take a truly neutral stance. Here, a neutral stance itself is an ideological stance. Any pose of strict neutrality is a masquerade. To view a change of religious frameworks as a potential means of therapy (for, say, Sisyphus) is itself a kind of ideology. In fact, it may well be an ideology that is peculiar to the late modern condition, a stance not unlike an academic class on comparative religion. (It is the stance that Stanley Hauerwas is gesturing toward when he says, "The project of modernity has been to produce people who believe they should have no story other than the story they chose when they had no story.")[10] This ideology, the therapeutic worldview, sees every human predicament as a problem to be fixed. (And if you disagree, that is probably because you are depressed.)

As Hauerwas points out, it is a mistake to blame the therapeutic worldview on doctors or psychiatrists or any other health care professionals. Every society gets the doctors it deserves, and our doctors are merely giving us what we demand. The language of sin and grace does not work for us anymore, or at least not for enough of us. Illness and treatment are the ways that we have come to understand our lives and our place in the universe. Even religion can be seen as a kind of therapy, an instrument to achieve spiritual comfort and psychic well-being. The therapeutic worldview has the additional advantage of allowing us to delegate knowledge and responsibility for our conditions as mortal beings to expert professionals. As Hauerwas puts it, "Patients have forgotten what every doctor knows, namely, that the final description for every patient for which a doctor cares is 'dead.'"[11]

But Kolakowski's spiritual conversion agency is also a satire of individualism, the myth of the self-contained, self-determining individual. To undergo a conversion like the ones that Kolakowski suggests would be impossible. A conversion could (in theory if not in actuality) bring about a change of belief and even a change in values, but our moral horizons are much broader than this. We cannot simply escape culture and history. We cannot simply create or discard the frameworks of meaning by which a life is judged meaningful or failed or wasted. We cannot fix everything simply by changing our own individual outlooks.

Yet the appeal of psychoactive medication depends on the premise that we can. Throughout much of the 1960s and 1970s the best-selling prescription drugs in America were Librium and Valium, the so-called minor tranquilizers. Doctors insisted that anxiety was a legitimate medical problem for which tranquilizers were a legitimate treatment, but this did not prevent Valium from becoming a symbol for the most soul-deadening aspects of American life. At one point in the 1970s, one in five American women was taking tranquilizers. Feminists responded, quite understandably, by asking, "With lives like that, who wouldn't need to be medicated?" Yet the feminist response misses the larger point. It is not hard to see why a 1970s suburban housewife would be alienated from a life devoted to laundry, soap operas, and shopping at the mall. But is this woman really going to be less alienated if she has a job in middle management, commutes to work every day, and spends her Saturdays perched on a riding mower? The point is not just that there is more to life than shopping and lawn care. The point is that it is possible for a person to be alienated from just about any kind of life. Do we see this alienation as a problem to be treated or as a sign that they might be onto something?

When Prozac came along in the wake of Valium's fall from grace, many people were tempted to see it in the same terms in which they saw Valium and Librium and, before them, Miltown: as emotional aspirin, as happiness pills, as yet another way of anesthetizing people against the sadness and anxiety of life in late twentieth-century America. Others insisted that, no, Prozac is different. It energizes rather than tranquilizes. It gives people confidence and self-esteem rather than a sense of relaxation. It produces long-term changes, not a quick fix. To a large degree these people were right. Yet the larger question remains. Is it always better for the anxious and alienated person to feel less anxious and alienated? Is there no other measure of a life other than a person's subjective sense of well-being? When a person says, as one man did on Prozac, "I don't have to look into the abyss anymore," is he or she necessarily better off? [12]

This is not just an abstract question. One of the lingering questions about Prozac and other SSRIs is the extent to which these drugs can blunt the sensitivity with which a person responds to the world around them, even as they improve that person's subjective sense of well-being. Some people who use the SSRIs, for example, find their social inhibitions loosened. This kind of loosening may well be one reason why the drugs are useful not just for depression but also for shyness, social phobia, and even (like Valium and Librium) for anxiety. They blunt the paralyzing self-consciousness that many Americans feel at the prospect of giving a presentation at a business meeting or making small talk at dinner parties. Yet sometimes a little self-consciousness is precisely what the circumstances call for. One early paper describes a thirty-five-year-old businesswoman who began taking an SSRI for panic disorder. At a company party, her friends had to prevent her from acting on her desire to serve cocktails to guests in her bra, "like Madonna."[13]

Other people find themselves disturbed by the extent to which the drugs narrow their ordinary emotional range. They do not worry as much, do not feel quite as lonely and fearful, do not experience grief with the same fierce intensity. This may be a blessing, of course, especially for people who are seriously depressed. But there is something deeply disconcerting about large sections of the population using medication to blunt their emotional responses to the world around them, and it is all the more disconcerting when the medication works so well and for so long. It is disconcerting not because of anything about a person's internal psychic state (Who doesn't want to be happier, less worried, less consumed with grief?) but because that internal psychic state does not match what the external world seems to be calling for. A fifty-year-old woman taking an SSRI says, "This must be what it feels like to have a lobotomy."[14]

I suspect that part of the worry many people have about Prozac has less to do with the drug itself than with the enthusiasm with which Americans in particular have embraced it. Why we have embraced it (apart from the merits of the drug itself, which are not at all inconsiderable) is a matter for speculation: a multibillion-dollar pharmaceutical industry, a native enthusiasm for technology, an ethic of competitive individualism, or a constitutional right to the pursuit of happiness. Yet along with that enthusiasm is the suspicion that psychopharmacology alone cannot account for the predicament in which we find ourselves, and that this predicament is not something that can be cured, as Wittgenstein says, with a medicine invented by an individual but, rather, by a change in our manner of living. And not by my own personal manner of living, or at least not solely, but by the way we all live now, together—by what Wittgenstein might call our form of life.

Of course, it may be that antidepressants will often cure depression without touching alienation, leaving a person alienated but not depressed. Whether this would be a good state to be in or not will depend on how you see our collective situation—whether, as Percy would say, you think we are in a predicament. Yet as long as we fail to take any account of these broader frameworks of significance, we cannot take account of alienation from them. Unless we think about meaning, we cannot take the measure of meaninglessness; unless we think about home, we cannot take the measure of homelessness; unless we recognize the fact of the journey, we cannot take account of the person who is lost. If, in Clifford Geertz's famous paraphrase of Max Weber, we are suspended in webs of significance that we ourselves have spun, then only by looking closely at how we are situated in those webs can we see how we may be trapped there, or falling, or gazing contentedly at the ceiling.

NOTES

1. Maureen O'Hara and Walter Truett Anderson, "Psychotherapy's Own Identity Crisis," in *The Fontana Postmodernism Reader*, ed. Walter Truett Anderson (London: Fontana Press, 1996), 166–67.

2. Alexis de Tocqueville, *Democracy in America* (1848), 12th ed., ed. J. P. Mayer, trans. George Lawrence (New York: Harper and Row, 1988), 536.

3. Ludwig Wittgenstein, *Remarks on the Foundations of Mathematics*, ed. G. E. Anscombe (Oxford: Basil Blackwell), 57.

4. Cornel West, *Race Matters* (Boston: Beacon Press, 1993), 15.

5. Walker Percy, *The Last Gentleman* (1966; reprint, London: Panther Books, 1985), 12.

6. Richard Ford, *Independence Day* (New York: Vintage, 1996), 57.

7. Walker Percy, *Love in the Ruins* (New York: Ivy Books, 1971), 12–13.

8. Walker Percy, *Signposts in a Strange Land*, ed. Patrick Samway (New York: Farrar, Straus and Giroux, 1991), 258.

9. Leszek Kolakowski, *Modernity on Endless Trial* (Chicago: University of Chicago Press, 1990), 120.

10. Stanley Hauerwas, "Sinsick," plenary address to the annual meeting of American Society of Bioethics and Humanities, Houston, Tex., November 1998.

11. Ibid.

12. Ronald W. Dworkin, "The Medicalization of Unhappiness," *Public Interest*, Summer 2001, 94.

13. Rudolf Hoehn-Saric, John R. Lipsey, and Daniel R. McLeod, "Apathy and Indifference in Patients on Fluvoxamine and Fluoxetine," *Journal of Clinical Psychopharmacology* 10, no. 5 (1990): 344–48. At the time, she saw this simply as "letting steam off," but once her Luvox dosage was decreased, she found her behavior inappropriate and "out of character."

14. Ibid., 344.

SECTION 3
Prozac and the East

SUSAN SQUIER

The Paradox of Prozac as an Enhancement Technology

For several years, two clippings have been taped to my filing cabinet. A *New Yorker* cartoon pictures two middle-aged women in a health club locker room, one saying to the other, "I've found that there are times in a person's spiritual journey when prescription drugs are entirely appropriate."[1] And a sentence cut from an advertisement for a CD-ROM promises, "In 28 minutes you'll be meditating like a Zen monk!" Both clippings address the relationship between enhancement technologies—"the use of medical technologies not to cure or control illness and disability but to enhance human capacities and characteristics"— and the spiritual realm.[2] Whether with humor or with reassurance, these clippings respond to the anxieties raised by the increasing social reliance on Prozac and other selective serotonin reuptake inhibitors (SSRIS). Are such prescription medications a dangerous flight from the authentic self? Do they substitute the comfort of accumulation (of things, of abilities and capacities) for the discomfort of facing social alienation and angst? Do these medications enable a form of spiritual "cheating": avoiding ultimate questions by engaging in a commodified form of self-fashioning? In what follows, I sidestep the either/or logic that structures these worries to suggest another way of thinking about Prozac as a way of life. I argue that despite the risks posed by its widespread commodification, Prozac can function as a *paradoxical* "less is more" enhancement technology. It can enhance human life not by amplification but by paring down, not by firming up identity but by fragmenting it, and not by aiding in the denial of death but by enabling its confrontation.

Let us begin with the *New Yorker* cartoon. While it articulates a recognizable masculinist scorn of women, together, taking themselves seriously, it is nonetheless funny because it invokes a number of different contemporary debates and discourses. We may laugh at fifty-something women engaging in lifestyle transformations; working with personal trainers, career coaches, and menopause groups; and participating in the growing movement of assertive body management that has come to be associated with "positive aging."[3] We may laugh at the ironic contrast between the experiences of these women with exercise and prescription drugs and the experimental forays of such mystical acidhead renegades as Timothy Leary, Ken Kesey, and Ram Dass. We may even laugh, if truth be told, because we assume that such well-ordered lives do not afford a spiritual dimension and such women do not embark on spiritual journeys. The tone of the cartoon's caption makes the same point with the measured impersonality of its language: what spiritual ecstasy or rebellion could fuel someone concerned with whether it is appropriate to use prescription drugs?

We do not know, of course, if the drug in the cartoon is Prozac or even another SSRI; it might be hormone replacement therapy (say, one of the new designer estrogens). But we know from the context that we are in the realm of psychological and physical *wellness* rather than illness. I begin with this cartoon, then, precisely because in addition to a gender-inflected subtext that I will ignore for the moment, it expresses some central anxieties about the social and spiritual implications of our society's increasing reliance on Prozac and the other SSRIS: that the medication is prescribed for frivolous reasons; that it is being taken by people to *improve* life rather than treat illness; that its ready availability produces a spiritual debasement, commodification, and diminution of life into *lifestyle*; and that it is prescribed far more widely to women than men, reflecting and perhaps perpetuating the problematic gender relations in our culture. In short, this cartoon reflects the assumption that Prozac is incompatible with authenticity and spirituality, and it depicts the fear that the medication can be used to reinforce, rather than to resist, oppressive cultural formations, from "workaholic" behavior to other-orientation. While I acknowledge the force of these anxieties, I question the specific constructions of life, death, and spirituality that are central to that model of authenticity.

As I will argue, we laugh at this cartoon for reasons intimately linked to our society of instrumental rationality and the particular spirituality it generates. In order to assess the meaning and potential of Prozac, we need to consider the relations that exist between our society and our spirituality, to imagine an alternative to our society of commodification and instrumentality, and to extrapolate from that alternative society an alternative spiritual life. Challenging the cartoon's implicit premise that spirituality is incompatible with certain kinds of embodied lives, we can come to an alternative understanding of the paradox of Prozac as an enhancement technology.

When Prozac is prescribed to make the user "better than well," its use arguably joins a set of behaviors that range from the medical to the social and personal. All are what sociologist Zygmunt Bauman calls "life strategies": the behaviors with which we deal with our awareness of mortality.[4] The process of managing mortality forms the core of all human societies, which by these activities transform the stark biological fact of death into the rich set of institutions, social formations, meanings, and behaviors that we know as culture. The range of these strategies is broad, but they all involve practical, pragmatic, specific practices that defensively refocus attention from the inevitability of death to the aversion of immediate, concrete threats to health.

In its attempt to cope with the knowledge of human mortality, Bauman argues, modern Western culture has turned to behaviors that offer the illusion of agency and control over life, thus making possible the (temporary) denial of death. "In the language of survival, practical concerns with specific dangers to life elbow out the metaphysical concern with death as the inescapable ending to existence."[5] A complex meld of social forces has given rise to this modern preoccupation with achieving short-term control over the problems of living: the declining authority of religious discourse, the dominance of a culture of expertise and rationality, the increasing isolation (and privatization) of dying and death, the increasing notion of the self and the body as a reflexive project, and the stress on achieving "a balance between opportunity and risk."[6] The convergence of these forces has led to a redirection of human effort in the modern West, away from generating meaning in a world to come and toward generating meaning today, in the here and now. While such a reorientation of meaning from the future to the present moment can be extremely valuable, in ways I will go on to discuss, all too often in the modern and postmodern eras these activities have taken on a particularly active, results-oriented, even compulsive quality. As Bauman observes, "Keeping fit, taking exercise, 'balancing the diet', eating fibres and not eating fat, avoiding smokers or fighting the pollution of drinking water are all feasible tasks, tasks that can be performed and that redefine the unmanageable problem (or, rather, non-problem) of death (which one can do nothing about) as a series of utterly manageable problems (which one can do something about; indeed, which one can do a lot about)."[7] Used in this context, enhancement technologies—from aromatherapy candles to psychotropic medications—offer a technological fix: they promise to produce freedom from illness, a sleeker or more athletic body, and ultimately a longer life.

These complex, collective, consumer-oriented body projects and life strategies are increasingly central to modernity because they offer ways of improving our selves and shaping the meaning of our lives. As Chris Shilling observes, in Western culture "there is a tendency for the body to be seen as an entity which is in the process of becoming; a project which should be worked at and accomplished as part of an *individual's* self-identity."[8] Moreover, as the *New Yorker* cartoon suggests, such deliberately shaped identities will also have a deliberately modified spirituality. Individual encounter with the large questions of life, mediated through religious experience, is replaced by a *spirituality* that is managed, controlled, tamed, and kept within bounds. Any exploration of life's ultimate meaning in the face of mortality is replaced by the attempt to delay death or reoriented toward exploration of specific practices to enhance or prolong human life, perhaps indefinitely. As exemplified by the books, videos, compact disks, and gift objects offered to subscribers by the One Spirit Book Club, a registered subsidiary of the Book-of-the-Month Club Inc., these highly marketable practices include body management routines generated by medical science (exercise, special diets, and techniques for managing insomnia) as well as para-scientific and para-spiritual cultural rituals for mind management (meditation, massage, and aromatherapy).[9]

When we do our Pilates, read Rumi, or surround ourselves with the aromatherapy candles and home altars featured in the feng shui guides we purchase from One Spirit, we manage our health and mitigate our risk of falling ill. Yet the bargain we make with such purchases is a mixed one. These self-reflexive activities raise a paradoxical question: even as we engage in them in order to extend life, are we somehow avoiding its essence? Or as Carl Elliott puts it, "At least part of the nagging worry about Prozac and its ilk is that for all the good they do, the ills that they treat are part and parcel of the lonely, forgetful, unbearably sad place where we live."[10]

PROZAC IS ZEN MEDICINE

Elliott's observation is crucial for our understanding of Prozac, but for reasons rather different from those he may have intended. I suggest that we may find a different answer to the nagging worry it articulates —that the SSRIs treat ills that are an inescapable part of the human condition—if we reexamine our notion of existence itself. What if we move beyond labeling that "place where we live," whether we label it as joyful or as "lonely, forgetful," and "unbearably sad"? An anecdote told by psychiatrist Mark Epstein suggests how relinquishing our assumptions about life—being open to an alternative perspective on the way we *expect* life to be—can also produce an alternative assessment of Prozac. Sally, a woman Epstein has seen for one consultation, calls him to ask his advice. After years of depression and anxiety, Sally has started taking Zoloft, one of the SSRIs, and has found significant relief. Now, however, she is about to leave for a two-week intensive meditation retreat, and she is afraid her medication will hamper her spiritual journey. As Epstein recalls, Sally feels uncomfortable about continuing her medication while on retreat: "Perhaps I should go more deeply into my problems while I'm away," Sally tells Epstein. She is concerned that the antidepressant would impede the process by making her problems less accessible to her. Epstein's response is decisive:

> I was relieved to hear that Sally was feeling better. People who respond well to these antidepressants often have few if any side effects. They find instead that they feel restored, healed of the depressive symptoms that they were expending so much of their energy trying to fend off. Less preoccupied with their internal states, they are freer to participate in their own lives, yet they often wonder if they are cheating. "This isn't the real me," they protest. "I'm the tired, cranky, no-good one you remember from a couple of weeks ago." As a psychiatrist, I am often in the position to encourage people to question those identifications. Depressed people think they know themselves, but maybe they only know depression.[11]

Distinguishing between "going into one's problems" and letting go of them in order to move in a new direction, Epstein encourages Sally to continue taking her medication because it is likely to assist her in the retreat. "I told her that at this point I felt she needed to come out of her problems, not go into them more deeply, and that the antidepressant should not get in her way in that regard. To be overwhelmed while on retreat would not be useful."[12]

This anecdote provides an alternative perspective on the two issues of pivotal importance in the debate over Prozac as an enhancement technology: the nature of a religious or spiritual encounter with life and the nature of identity. Sally's sense that the medicine would hamper her spiritual inquiry by making her "calmer, less irritable, and . . .

happier" begs the first question: is spiritual inquiry inherently upsetting and painful? In a discussion of the spiritual implications of Prozac use, Tod Chambers challenges the conventional understanding that Prozac is used as a pharmacological bandage on spiritual angst. Instead, he proposes that such an argument relies on a one-sided view of religious experience as motivated primarily by suffering. As an alternative to this, he offers William James's more complex formulation of the two types of religious temperaments: the "sick soul" and "healthy mindedness."[13] Both temperaments are on display, Chambers argues, in Lauren Slater's *Prozac Diary*. Having suffered from severe psychiatric impairments her whole life, Slater achieves a remarkable recovery when she starts taking Prozac. The effect extends beyond the relief of psychiatric symptoms to a dramatic reordering of her philosophical and spiritual worlds. While Slater had always been drawn to the melancholy philosophical writings of Søren Kierkegaard and Victor Frankl, after treatment with Prozac she finds herself more interested in the contemplative works of Thomas Merton.

Her religious perspective has shifted, but it has not disappeared. This crucial fact complicates any argument that Prozac replaces spirituality with complacency, suffering with ersatz, pharmacologically induced happiness. Instead, Slater is exploring a new kind of spirituality. As she explains, Prozac has opened her up to the beauty of life in the moment: "We who are permanently camped here see things you don't see at 55 mph."[14] Instead of life in the fast lane, with its emphasis on the passage of time and the agony of impending mortality, Slater finds herself "camped" in one place, newly attuned to the richness of each moment of life. "This is the real problem with Prozac. As I stay on it longer . . . I am discovering that, like a pair of parentheses, it brackets back the noisy numbness, the staccato pricks of panic. Prozac is Zen medicine, and taking it, I find myself a Zen novitiate, a Trappist oblate, trying to learn some spiritual tradition I have no knack for. Because, surely, there must be something sacred in the quiet quotidian that illness has caused me to miss."[15]

As Slater describes her experience, Prozac has exposed her to an alternative spiritual mode, one closer to Eastern religious practices and unfamiliar to most people who have grown up in Western religions, except the contemplative Christianity of the Trappists. She has shifted her focus from the attempt to control the future to attempts to experience the present—"attempts," because both tradition and training make such a reorientation of perspective quite difficult. Indeed, Slater suggests that to one raised in the Jewish or conventional Christian traditions, this new focus on the "quiet quotidian" even seems "a conduit to sin" because it shifts one's attention from the transcendent to those "tasks, the tiny things, altogether less transcendent."[16] Prozac seems potentially sinful to her because it challenges the teleological foundations of Judeo-Christian society with an alternative investment in the here and now.

Slater draws on a range of sensory metaphors to express the visceral impact of her new experience. No longer preoccupied with "the grand and deep darkness," now she lives "in the daily light, slowly learning to see its spectrum."[17] As she explains, the change also registers in tactile and auditory ways. The medication sets her free from relentless hearing, so she is now for the first time able to "decode silence." "In the long run, the cure called Prozac doesn't fill your mind so much as empty it of its contents and then leave you, like a pitcher, waiting to be filled."[18] This new access to emptiness and silence, this slow attentiveness to the everyday, suggests that medication gives Slater both a new mode of spirituality and a model for identity.

What does Slater mean when she refers to "the problem with Prozac?" In what sense does it stem from its status as "Zen medicine"? The altered sense of time, in which things can develop at their own pace rather than being forced; the awareness of silence; and the shift in focus from the transcendent to the immanent, from the permanent to the evanescent, will be familiar to anyone who practices Zen Buddhist meditation. The techniques of *zazen*, motionless sitting meditation; *shikan-taza*, the Zen practice of "just sitting" without a goal; and *kinhin*, extremely slow walking meditation, train one to quiet the mind, focus on the breath, and watch one's thoughts without either identifying with them or attempting to control them.

What is the result of such meditation? Rather than shoring up that solid, bounded, impervious sense of self foundational to Western rationalism, meditation introduces the practitioner to the concept of emptiness. But to paraphrase the Zen student in another *New Yorker* cartoon, "What is this emptiness I've been hearing so much about?"[19] Emptiness is a difficult concept for persons trained philosophically to affirm the autonomy of things and to uphold the subject/object distinction. Rather than meaning nonexistence, emptiness means interdependence, impermanence, transcendence of the very notions of self and other. As Epstein explains, "Emptiness (or *sunyata*), from a Buddhist perspective, [is] an understanding of one's true nature, an intuition of the absence of inherent identity in people or in things."[20] Zen master Sekito Kisen put it this way in the eighth-century poem known as "The Sandokai": "Things and emptiness are like a container and its cover fitting together / like two arrows meeting head-on."[21]

In fact, to talk about *zazen* or *shikan-taza* as having a result is to miss the point, for goal orientation is the first quality a practitioner of meditation relinquishes (again and again) along with notions of a stable core self and of life as a race. Slater labels her experience with Prozac as a spiritual one, linking it to Zen and Trappist meditative practices, because it introduces a view of life and society diametrically opposed to the life strategies of those *New Yorker* cartoon women, who rely on their health club workouts and prescription medications to control aging and deny death. Rather than responding to emptiness with denial or a panicky shoring up of the self, the meditator learns to tolerate the experience of emptiness, even to affirm it.

The problem with Prozac? Consider what it would mean to put into practice the insights generated by this alternative experience. Rather than letting our ontological insecurity propel us into engaging in all the varied body projects of modernity, what would happen if we were instead to confront that insecurity and acknowledge its fundamental reality? What would happen if we acknowledged the impermanence that is so central to having a mortal body? What would the outcome be if we stopped busying ourselves—with exercise, cosmetics, vitamins, and all such forms of antiaging work—and began to attend to the shifting ground on which we stand? What would happen if we stopped our high-speed consumption and instead simply slowed down and lived each moment? Such a shift, if made on a large scale, could have economic as well as psychological and social implications. Certainly, it would jeopardize the expanding self-care industry. Even on a small scale that shift in perspective could catalyze disengagement from the risk society of late modernity. Why focus on more, better, faster, when now is all we have? Perhaps it is reasonable to be alienated from a society in which attempts at risk management are the only available models for responding to the fundamental impermanence of life. Still, for the machinery of that society, from risk management to health care and lifestyle enhancement strategies, the new perspective enabled by Prozac could indeed be destabilizing.

Yet there is a contradiction here, or perhaps several. First, Prozac not only undercuts but participates in the system of social organization and self-understanding from which it has arisen: the "reflexive encounter with expert systems helping to reconstitute the self [that] therefore expresses some of the central dilemmas to which modernity gives rise."[22] Because Prozac use is initiated on the advice of a physician or psychiatrist who must prescribe the drug, which is made available by the pharmacological industry, it is also embedded in the precise system of technical expertise, commodity production, and scientific rationality that I have been arguing it stands to threaten. Moreover, Prozac use can be marketed as an easy solution to the contradictions and pains of our culture, producing peaceful adolescents in a society discouraging rebellion, docile workers in a class-stratified society, and "happy" women and people of color in a sexist, racist culture. Whether we understand Prozac as a good solution to the problem of depression or a bad solution to the problem of domestic violence (because it medicates the woman into remaining in an oppressive relationship), in either case we are viewing the medication as the solution in a problem-solution logic. Because this is a logic that reproduces itself endlessly, proliferating good Prozac/bad Prozac debates, it distracts us from another, more productive mode of encountering Prozac: not as an essence but as a set of practices. Even here, the otherworldly earnestness characterizing the meditative life lived *in the moment* (to the mantra "No day but today") is undercut by its familiarity as a highly profitable lifestyle. These centering practices are much more likely to decenter, for they are marketed not only by the publishing industry (the One Spirit Book Club and the jarringly titled *Real Simple*, the new century's answer to *Self* magazine) but by the music industry, too (witness the blockbuster Broadway musical *Rent* and its successful CD), to create consumer desire.

Perhaps because the contradiction at the heart of Prozac use is also present at the heart of Western Zen Buddhism, I find in Zen logic a way out of the either/or impasse that has dominated our cultural response to it. Buddhism, like Prozac, is currently a hot commodity, generating merchandise (*zafus*, Zen books, and incense sticks), experiences (a Roshi-led trip to sacred Eastern sites, or a star-studded conference on contemporary Buddhism), and even new corporate strategies (teaching contemplative practices to Monsanto executives). But such commodification poses great contradictions for Buddhist practice, David Patt argues in an article in *Tricycle: The Buddhist Review*: "Any marketing wizard will tell you that fast and easy enlightenment will sell better than banging your head on the ground."[23]

Now that advertisements promote the curative effects of meditation, the spiritual impact of Buddhist tourism, and the appeal of luxury Zen retreats ("Indulge Yourself," one ad exhorts), is there an increasing tendency to emphasize the comfortable and appealing aspects of Buddhist practice over its rigors? And what are the implications of this for spiritual practice? Are the compromises involved in marketing Buddhism acceptable within a Zen perspective? "Is it the case, then, that Buddhism commodified is Buddhism lite, Buddhism with a happy face?"[24] Patt's answer to this difficult question (one that parallels the concern about the inauthentic happiness that Prozac can purvey) is to counsel the middle way: an embrace of the contemporary technologies of marketing, tempered by a self-reflexive examination of the possible social cost of such methods.[25]

The way I have been thinking about Prozac so far entails walking out of that problem-solution logic. Rather than attempting to judge whether Prozac is a good or a bad solution to a problem, I suggest we stop categorizing experience into problems and solutions and stop automatically assuming that commodification is—at best—a necessary evil. Instead, we might turn our attention to what Shunryu Suzuki called "things-as-it-is" as distinct from "things-as-they-are."

> Suzuki Roshi also made up phrases of his own in order to express himself in a more non-dualistic way. For instance, he often used the phrase "things-as-it-is" to mean the fundamental nature of reality, something beyond words. But he also used "things-as-they-are" to refer to our usual discriminating, dualistic way of thinking and perceiving (good/bad, right/wrong). He was well aware of the difference. In "things-as-it-is," his use of the singular and plural in the same phrase stretches our ordinary way of thinking.[26]

Perhaps we need a similar stretch in our ordinary way of thinking about the complex molecule that comprise(s) Prozac and the complex identity that is (are) the self. Zen logic, with its rejection of binaries and its skepticism about essences, can reveal the paradoxical malleability of Prozac as an enhancement technology. Like Zen itself, Prozac can be (and often is) commodified. But we can learn from Donna Haraway that commodities—like cyborgs—are not always faithful to their origins.[27] Considering an even more suspect commodity, the Barbie doll, we can learn from J. K. Gibson-Graham, an author who herself puts into crisis the notion of a unitary identity, that "the market is not all or only capitalist, commodities are not all or only products of capitalism, and the sale of Barbie dolls to Indian girls or boys does not at all or only presage the coming of the global heterosexist capitalist kingdom."[28] The commodity form of Prozac obviously comes as a solution at the conjunction of a great many problem-solution logics, but that does not mean that Prozac will always and everywhere function in ways that are true to that origin.

Indeed, recent experience teaches us that neither will Zen Buddhism itself. *The Shoes outside the Door*, Michael Downing's exploration of the 1983 scandals at the San Francisco Zen Center, traces the unpredictable events that followed Shunryu Suzuki's installation of Richard Baker as the chief priest, or head abbot, of the first Western Zen Buddhist monastery. The series of sexual, economic, and psychological missteps that characterized Baker's tenure in the "Mountain Seat," hotly debated though they were and no doubt continue to be, without any doubt constituted unpredictable and unskillful wandering from the path of Zen. Yet as Suzuki biographer David Chadwick relates, in another way they *were* predicted, albeit ironically, by one of Suzuki's last statements to his wife: "I won't interfere with Zen Center at all once I have handed it over to Richard. It's entirely up to him whether it will be ruined or not."[29] "What is the true meditation?" Zen Master Hakuin asked. "It is to make everything: coughing, swallowing, waving the arms, motion, stillness, words, action, the evil and the good, prosperity and shame, gain and loss, right and wrong, into one single koan."[30]

FROM *EREWHON* TO ELECTRIC ZEN

This brings me to the second clipping on my filing cabinet: "In 28 minutes you'll be meditating like a Zen monk!" I love the absurd paradox in the advertisement: the notion that something so rigorous and spare as Zen meditation could be made effortless and speedy through technological mediation. Even longer than the use of medications to relieve depression, the application of technical enhancement to the practice of *zazen* has been the subject of much debate within Zen Buddhist thought. Because these debates turn on the questions of identity, agency, and control, they can also illuminate the paradoxical role of Prozac as an enhancement technology. Understood (and positioned) as neither a sin nor a sophisticated medical treatment but as a neutral commodity, the electric version of Zen, available via CD-ROM, promises to induce a hard-to-achieve brain wave frequency, accelerate the process of meditation, and thus give its user a competitive edge on the old-fashioned, low-tech methods of the Zen monk. Though the commodification of this practice as part of the entertainment industry (along with New Age healing CDs and videos) is relatively new, the technique of biofeedback-based acceleration to meditation has been around for more than a quarter-century as a medical practice. Arguably, such varied forms of technological intervention, whether mechanical, medical, chemical, or electronic, migrate over time from the illicit to the medical and, finally, to the commercial and commodified.[31] Is there a difference between them? If the chemical intervention of Prozac can enable access to the celebration of the quiet quotidian, what about the electrical intervention of biofeedback? Does it enable a shortcut to Zen enlightenment?

An exchange between Philip Kapleau, the author of one of the most important early explorations of Zen Buddhism for a Western audience, and a questioner at one of his intensive retreats in 1978 clarifies the differences between regular *zazen* and what Kapleau calls electric Zen:

> QUESTIONER: I read somewhere that brain-wave feedback will bring the same results after just a few weeks or months that requires years of effort in Zen.
>
> ROSHI [laughing]: You must be kidding! To claim that spiritual awakening and a transformation of personality can be accomplished at all—let alone more quickly—simply by hooking up to a machine is ridiculously naïve. Even if one is able while "plugged in" to ease into a relaxed state, this hardly brings deep calm or lasting peace of mind; it does not answer fundamental questions of existence; it does not transform one's life in any real way, all of which Zen awakening does. . . . One who regularly plugs into a machine to relax loses the ability to act out of his or her own deepest resources and instead of being master of the machine becomes a slave.[32]

Roshi Kapleau's objections to electric Zen raise the issues that predominate in all discussions of enhancement technology, whether electronic, mechanical, or chemical: control, agency, and identity. A decade before Prozac hit the market, Kapleau articulated the main concerns that would arise in response. In surrendering control and agency to technology, do human beings gain the chance to improve their situation (by relaxing, for example), only to lose the ability decisively to transform their identities?

The anxiety that machines can control human beings dates back at least to Samuel Butler's *Erewhon* (1872), the satire of a society that has banned all machines out of fear that they might take the upper hand. As Butler's narrator worries, "May not man himself become a sort of parasite upon the machines?"[33] The human use of machinery seems to threaten spirituality itself: "Man's very soul is due to the machines;

it is a machine-made thing; he thinks as he thinks, and feels as he feels, through the work that machines have wrought upon him, and their existence is quite as much as *sine qua non* for his, as his for theirs." Yet as Butler's narrator defends the use of machinery, he leads us to see the danger in its use (whether the technology is mechanical, chemical, or electrical): "True, from a low materialistic point of view, it would seem that those thrive best who use machinery wherever its use is possible with profit; but this is the art of the machines—they serve that they may rule. . . . They have preyed upon man's groveling preferences for his material over his spiritual interests."[34] The narrator's fear that human control could be ceded to machines beyond the self is not the only worry, however; he also fears *chemical* technologies. In a striking anticipation of our contemporary debate about psychopharmacology, the narrator wonders whether "every sensation is not chemical and mechanical in its operation? Whether those things which we deem most purely spiritual are anything but disturbances of equilibrium."[35] In other words, he raises the possibility that human control could be lost not to something outside the self but to something *within* it, here conceptualized as a chemical imbalance. Thus, a century before Prozac and biofeedback, in *Erewhon* a prescient Samuel Butler raised the question, Is human identity itself chemical and mechanical?

While Butler wrote from the perspective of skeptical Christianity, the critique he raised in 1872 concerning the human reliance on machines reappeared a century later in the questions that Buddhists raised about biofeedback, and then again at the turn of the twenty-first century in debates within Buddhism about the uses of psychopharmacology, and the SSRIs in particular. In a searching discussion titled "Prozac and the Enlightened Mind," Judith Hooper traces the evolving response within the Buddhist community to the question raised in the *New Yorker* cartoon: Can prescription medication be appropriate for a spiritual journey? A shift has occurred, Hooper argues. Only a decade ago, or perhaps less, students of Buddhism suffering from depression would be counseled by their Roshi to meditate harder. Now, Buddhist practitioners are increasingly open to the value of antidepressants, while there has been a surge of interest in the effects of meditation on the neurotransmitters. The Dalai Lama has participated in studies of his brain activity while meditating; neuroscientist James H. Austin, himself a practitioner of Zen meditation, has published a massive study of Zen and the brain; and psychiatrist Paul Fleischman announced to Hooper, "I feel emboldened to say that vipassana meditation changes your neurotransmission."[36]

This new tempered acceptance of psychopharmacology may reflect the influence of psychotherapist and Zen practitioner Philip Martin, whose book *The Zen Path through Depression* maps out what could be described as the middle way on Prozac use. Martin eschews both the enslavement to technology that Butler's characters feared in the nineteenth century and Kapleau feared in the 1970s and the angst-based construction of spirituality linked to our society of technoscientific rationality. Instead of looking to the future for a hoped-for control or the promise of ultimate meaning, Martin argues, we need to reorient our attention to the present moment. To put it another way, he maintains that we need to use medication, like the other techniques for addressing depression, not as life strategies through which we avoid the bitter truths of life but as centering techniques through which we can encounter them.

> We may expect that because of therapy, dietary changes, or medication, our depression will end. We hope for positive results—maybe even enlightenment—from our meditation. Yet all of this is about the future. When we are caught up in the future, we are no longer present with what we are doing right now, but looking ahead to the results. . . . If we use meditation or some other spiritual practice to obtain something, to improve or advance ourselves in some way, then we are using it as we use everything else in our lives. It is just like the expensive car, the right clothes, the right relationship, and all those things that we hope will bring us happiness in some future moment.[37]

A dense and important distinction is at work here, between understanding any enhancement technology (including Prozac) as a means and thinking of it as an end. Enhancement technologies can be useful as ways of producing an atmosphere for work, but they are not substitutes for the work itself. As Kapleau points out, electric Zen cannot substitute for genuine encounter with the fundamental questions of existence, and if used that way, it would clearly represent a form of spiritual cheating. But what does this tell us about the role Prozac can play in Zen Buddhist meditation? Let us return to the case of Mark Epstein's patient, Sally. Struggling with a depression, Sally would be most likely to make good use of her *sesshin* (intensive meditation retreat), Epstein explains, if she continues her medication. She can thus use the SSRI to reduce internal noise and lift the burden of her cycling depressive thoughts, thus gaining access to the meditative experience that is her goal. The medication can actually increase Sally's *agency*, so that she can actively engage in her meditation practice. In fact, meditation is paradoxically both a means toward what Kapleau calls a spiritual awakening and the awakening itself. As Zen Master Dogen puts it, "The practice of meditation is not a method for the attainment of realization—it is enlightenment itself."[38]

Unlike the instantaneous result afforded by electric Zen, Kapleau argues that "years of effort in Zen" can bring about a "transformation of personality." His comment returns us from the issues of agency and control to the fundamental question of identity, and to the *New Yorker* cartoon of the women in the health club. Despite the cartoon, which mocks the notion of spiritual experiences as incongruous for the middle-class, middle-aged health club members it pictures, I do understand Prozac as compatible with a certain kind of spiritual journey. When it is used to enable the goalless sitting, the *stillness* of meditation, medication can give rise to a fundamentally different notion of identity. Unlike the enhancement technologies or life strategies by which we shore up (in fantasy at least) a solid, unitary, permanent identity, meditation is closer to a practice, a kind of play, that dissolves identity. The practice of Zen meditation made possible by SSRIs is grounded in the understanding that "to be empty is not to be nonexistent. It is to be without a permanent identity. . . . The notion of *emptiness*, according to Buddhism, is therefore the affirmation of the existence of things and not their negation. Our desire for a world in which things are permanent and indestructible is neither realizable nor desirable."[39] Mark Epstein describes the spiritual insight that can be enabled by such an encounter with the dissolution of identity, in vivid contrast to the habitual modernist solidification of self: "Self-development, self-esteem, self-confidence, self-expression, self-awareness, and self-control are our most sought after attributes. But Buddhism teaches us that happiness does not come from any kind of acquisitiveness, be it material or psychological. Happiness comes from letting go. In Buddhism, the impenetrable, separate, and individuated self is more of the problem than the solution."[40]

TELLING TIME

Achieving happiness by letting go: the notion is in striking contrast to the anxious shoring up of health and self in response to mortality. How can such a process of surrender be life enhancing? Let me turn from the cartoon and the advertisement to a dream:

I am taking my usual exercise walk with my husband when my wristwatch falls off, its glass face breaking open when it hits the sidewalk. A cockroach crawls out; its carapace has cracked and it oozes thick yellow fluid. I am alarmed, and say I want to go into the Asian Market to buy some soy. "Now you're just going to have to tell time like the rest of us," my husband says.

I had this dream four years ago, about two months after recovering from major surgery. Intense abdominal pain had plagued me for some time; when my doctor finally discovered the ovarian mass, she moved quickly to perform a hysterectomy-ovariectomy. Surgery catapulted me, unwillingly and suddenly, into the realm of the postmenopausal. I had always been very active: walking, taking exercise classes, and swimming. I was a regular in the locker room of the university natatorium, and I took pride in my increasing strength and staying power. The illness and surgery were a huge shock; I felt betrayed by my body, no longer strong and energetic, but weak, tired, and old. Worse, I was no longer fertile. Before surgery, at age forty-seven, I had thought occasionally of having one more child. My sudden, surgically induced menopause had made that no longer possible. The ovary, my time-piece since puberty, had been removed. It was spoiled, broken, cradling not an ovum but a pus-filled cockroach.

The dream captures what was, for me, a traumatic experience: a painful illness, succeeded by surgery and the challenge of recuperation. Because surgery produced sudden menopause, my surgeon put me on hormone replacement therapy. This was a disappointment, too; like many women in my cohort, I had hoped to have a *natural* menopause. I tried to cut the hormone dosage in half and began a whole range of health-enhancement practices. I bought soy milk, flax seed, and tofu. The hot flashes and other discomforts continued. I recommenced my exercise routine and tried to get back to teaching and writing. But the loss of my old cycle had shaken more than my reproductive identity. "Now you're just going to have to tell time like the rest of us," my husband says to me in the dream. I began to do more than just tell time; I became obsessed with time's passing, obsessed with aging. Again, the dream documents how the temporal contours of my world had changed. I was forced to acknowledge the limits on my control over the passage of time, whether technologies of the self (exercise and special diets) or mechanical technologies (like my watch).

I went into a profound depression. Not that I knew it was depression at first. I just felt I had lost control of my body, my mind, and my life. No more brisk exercise walking; now it felt like I was walking through molasses. I could not sleep, could not concentrate, and could not remember things. Teaching was difficult. I forgot the ends of my sentences, forgot students' names, lost confidence, and tripped over myself apologizing for inadequacies. Writing became excruciating. Either my thoughts cycled repeatedly or they ground to a halt as I stared at the computer screen. I cried frequently; the tears would start for no reason, and I would be unable to stop them. I obsessively criticized myself or I felt flat, becalmed, and numb. I could not see where my life was going next. As I sat in my study, gazing across the beautiful meadow to the mountain above it, my eyes were turned inward, gazing on a landscape that was gray, barren, and dry. Into the realm of expert consultations and self-technologies I went: I consulted a psychiatrist, and she prescribed Prozac.

I knew the medication was working within two weeks. One day, my mind seemed quieter. The self-denigrating, guilty, hopeless thoughts were gone. Not that they stopped immediately, as if a switch had been turned off; rather, they just gradually lost their force. The pain I was carrying around me—a fog between me and the world—receded. My family, my life, and myself: I was enjoying them all once more. Life seemed to be moving again. But even with the depression under control, I told my psychiatrist, I still felt a hollowness at the core of life: a loss. A Quaker, she understood what I was describing. She knew that this was an experience I needed not to control or to defend against, but to encounter.[41] Had I ever tried meditation, she asked? Not since college, when I had written a paper comparing Zen and Christian meditative poetry. But I gave it a try.

For the first time in nearly thirty years, I began to meditate. Over the next several years, I found that the meditation and the medication worked together to allow me to experience myself differently. The Prozac enabled me, over time, to sit still and to tolerate the intense and sometimes painful feelings that emerged in meditation. Rather than working to shore up the illusion of physical and psychological invulnerability that had been so badly shaken by my illness and surgery, I began in meditation to sit with the feelings that had impinged so frighteningly with my illness. Instead of focusing only on what I had lost (on illness, on aging), I began to have tiny glimpses of the interconnectedness of things, the limitless pleasures in one moment, the joys of each new spring. I started gardening and found a *zendo*—a center for Soto Zen practice—near my house, where I could attend daylong gatherings as well as an occasional *sesshin*, or intensive meditation retreat.

A *zendo* in central Pennsylvania? That initially seems as incongruous as describing the experience of the last five years as a spiritual journey. Perhaps that is one of the paradoxes I have been writing about. There is another, too: like American Zen Buddhism, Prozac can be both a disturbingly decentering, profit-generating cultural commodity *and* a useful vehicle for one's spiritual journey. To adapt a line from *The Sopranos*: Spirituality, like hope, comes in many forms. I am reminded of the Zen parable about attachment: A pilgrim on a journey came to a raging river and made himself a raft to cross it. Once he reached the other side, he picked up the raft, put it on his head, and prepared to continue his pilgrimage. His traveling companion asked, "You needed the raft to cross the torrent, but why do you take it with you now that you're on the other side?" In the last year, I have stopped taking the Prozac. I continue to practice *zazen*.

NOTES

1. *New Yorker*, February 14, 2000, 74.

2. Carl Elliott, *A Philosophical Disease: Bioethics, Culture, and Identity* (New York: Routledge, 1998), 27.

3. For an example, see *The Positive Aging Newsletter*, compiled by Ken and Mary Gergen, <http://www.healthandage.com>.

4. Zygmunt Bauman, *Mortality, Immortality, and Other Life Strategies* (Stanford: Stanford University Press, 1992), 9.

5. Ibid., 130.

6. Anthony Giddens, *Modernity and Self-Identity: Self and Society in the Late Modern Age* (Stanford: Stanford University Press, 1991), 78. I am also drawing here on Bauman, *Mortality*, and Ulrich Beck, *Risk Society: Towards a New Modernity* (London: Sage, 1992).

7. Bauman, *Mortality*, 130.

8. Chris Shilling, *The Body and Social Theory* (London: Sage, 1993), 5.

9. *One Spirit Review*, January 2002.

10. Carl Elliott, "Pursued by Happiness and Beaten Senseless: Prozac and the American Dream," *Hastings Center Report* 30, no. 2 (2000): 8.

11. Mark Epstein, *Going on Being: Buddhism and the Way of Change* (New York: Broadway Books, 2001), 3–4.

12. Ibid., 6.

13. Tod Chambers, "Should the Buddha Have Taken Prozac? Religious Implications of SSRIs," *Park Ridge Center Bulletin*, January/February 2001, 5–6.

14. Lauren Slater, *Prozac Diary* (New York: Penguin, 1998), 85.

15. Ibid., 81.

16. Ibid., 89.

17. Ibid., 78.

18. Ibid.

19. The original caption reads, "Exactly what is this 'nothing' I've been hearing so much about?," *New Yorker*, July 31, 2000.

20. Epstein, *Going on Being*, 13.

21. "The Sandokai," compiled translation by Shunryu Suzuki, in *Branching Streams Flow in the Darkness: Zen Talks on the Sandokai*, by Shunryu Suzuki (Berkeley: University of California Press, 1999), 191.

22. Giddens, *Modernity and Self-Identity*, 143.

23. David Patt, "Who's Zoomin' Who? The Commodification of Buddhism in the American Marketplace," *Tricycle*, Summer 2001, esp. 44, 91.

24. Ibid., 91.

25. For a fascinating consideration of the implications of bringing Buddhist meditation to corporate culture, see Helen Tworkov's interview with Mirabai Bush, "Contemplating Corporate Culture," in *Tricycle*, Summer 2001, esp. 83.

26. Mel Weitsman, introduction to Suzuki, *Branching Streams Flow in the Darkness*, 7–8.

27. "The main trouble with cyborgs, of course, is that they are the illegitimate offspring of militarism and patriarchal capitalism. . . . But illegitimate offspring are often exceedingly unfaithful to their origins" (Donna Haraway, "A Cyborg Manifesto: Science, Technology, and Socialist-Feminism in the Late Twentieth Century," in *Simians, Cyborgs, and Women: The Reinvention of Nature* [New York: Routledge, 1991], 151). Thanks to Evan Watkins for his comments on this essay.

28. J. K. Gibson-Graham, *The End of Capitalism (as we knew it): A Feminist Critique of Political Economy* (Oxford: Blackwell, 1996), 144.

29. David Chadwick, *Crooked Cucumber: The Life and Zen Teaching of Shunryu Suzuki* (New York: Broadway Books, 1945), 401.

30. Judith Blackstone and Zoran Josipovic, *Zen for Beginners* (New York: Writers and Readers, 1986), 121.

31. For a discussion of the migration of another set of enhancement technologies from illicit pseudoscience to legitimate medicine, see Susan Squier, "Incubabies and Rejuvenates: The Traffic between Technologies of Reproduction and Age-Extension," in *Figuring Age: Women, Bodies, Generations*, ed. Kathleen Woodward (Bloomington: Indiana University Press, 1999), 88–111.

32. Philip Kapleau, *Zen: Merging of East and West* (1978; reprint, New York: Anchor Books, 2000), 42.

33. Samuel Butler, *Erewhon* (1872; reprint, New York: Penguin Classics, 1985), 206.

34. Ibid., 206–7.

35. Ibid., 201.

36. James H. Austin, M.D., *Zen and the Brain* (Cambridge, Mass.: MIT Books, 1999); Judith Hooper, "Prozac and the Enlightened Mind," *Tricycle*, Summer 1999, 109.

37. Philip Martin, *The Zen Path through Depression* (San Francisco: Harper, 1999), 103–4.

38. Zen Master Dogen, "Practice of Meditation [adapted from the *Fukanzazengi* by Senzaki and McCandless]," *Teachings of the Buddha*, ed. Jack Kornfield (Boston: Shambhala, 1996), 150.

39. Thich Nhat Hanh, *Zen Keys: A Guide to Zen Practice* (1973; reprint, New York: Doubleday, 1995), 106–7.

40. Mark Epstein, *Going to Pieces without Falling Apart: A Buddhist Perspective on Wholeness* (New York: Broadway Books, 1998), xvi.

41. Surveying women's Prozac narratives, Jonathan Metzl, in "Prozac and the Pharmacokinetics of Narrative Form," *Signs: Journal of Women in Culture and Society* 27, no. 2 (2001): 347–80, has argued that they are characterized by a problematic triple movement. First, the narrative repudiates the historicist, depth-oriented, lack-based model of female subjectivity deployed by psychoanalysis in favor of a biologically based, presentist, non-gender-binarized model of female agency. However, the biologically based escape from "the gendered weight of the psychoanalytic paradigm" is short lived, for the crisis known as the "Prozac poop-out" allows the narrative subject's psychological symptoms (depression, obsessive-compulsive disorder) to re-emerge (366). Now she is forced to acknowledge the limitations of the pharmacologically induced experience of agency that she had previously celebrated. The logic of control, agency, self-presence, and self-determination found in the refusal of psychoanalysis with its theory based on lack is thus lost when the narrator reencounters her contingent, abject, and symptom-producing self. Finally, she rebels also against that biologically based model of the self, affirming instead a self beyond both gendered neuroses and biologized self-determination. As the narrator affirms a self beyond both the lack-based model of psychoanalysis and the biologically based model of Prozac, however, she is paradoxically still taking the medication. As Metzl points out, this doubled return to a biological solution for what are supra-biological problems brackets the liberation the Prozac narrator asserts: "Prozac works to break down a binary, but at the same time it serves to ensure that the binary remains intact. The Prozac of liberation is also, ironically, the Prozac of the return of the repressed" (377). Wondering, as I read Metzl's essay, how

SUSAN SQUIER

my narrative corresponds to the category of Prozac narratives he describes, I have concluded that it diverges with the turn to *zazen*. While the essence of the biologized self (and the Cartesian self that, as Metzl points out, it reinstates) is its refusal of the unconscious, the abject, the transcient, and the contingent, all of those aspects of experience comprise the "three kinds of suffering" to which *zazen* opens one: the suffering of pain, the suffering of change, and the suffering of conditionality.

LAURENCE J. KIRMAYER

The Sound of One Hand Clapping
Listening to Prozac in Japan

INTRODUCTION: PSYCHOPHARMACOLOGY
IN THE GLOBAL VILLAGE

New psychopharmacological agents offer the prospect of regulating dysphoric moods among many people who were formerly viewed as having temperamental or character traits that rendered them shy, inhibited, or melancholic. Some of these people state they "feel like a new person" or, more paradoxically, that they have finally found their real or true selves. How are we to judge transformations of the self that are caused by drugs? Is a more functional self or happier self more real? Does our "true" self have any meaning other than the self we prefer and endorse or that others agree to hold us to?

Critics have raised the prospect of a "cosmetic psychopharmacology,"[1] applied like makeup to make us look *and* feel good, while our existential predicaments go unanswered. What if it is true that we now have the chemical technology to reconfigure our brains, to "sculpt our personalities,"[2] to make ourselves more outgoing, gregarious, bold, and optimistic? Should we not all drink the potion that will make us larger selves? If we feel some trepidation, how does the use of this technology differ practically or ethically from the many disciplines of the self—ancient and modern—aimed at refining our character?[3]

This debate takes place against a backdrop of cultural assumptions about the nature of depression, emotion, personality, and the good life. In this essay I try to lay bare and challenge some of these assumptions through considering the relative lack of use of antidepressants in Japan until very recently. This cultural difference may be a temporary anomaly related to the history of psychiatry and the local development of widely available mental health services. Within Japan, as in every country, there is wide variation in belief and practice among clinicians and laypeople. Cultural change is also occurring at an extraordinarily rapid pace through the forces of globalization, so that any characterization of a cultural world is likely to be outdated by the time it is committed to print. Nevertheless, national and cultural differences in psychiatric practice—however quickly they fade in response to market forces and the transfer of knowledge and technology —raise some basic questions about what it is that we treat when we give antidepressant medication.

I will explore the relevance for bioethics of cultural variations in the use of antidepressants at three different levels of analysis: (1) the varieties of depressive experience as they unfold in specific cultural worlds and value systems, (2) the narrative construction of the self, and (3) the political economic context of the pharmacological treatment of depression. Important ethical issues reside in the links between these levels. The strong interconnections of values framed at one level with those at other levels mean that there are likely to be unavoidable tradeoffs between different values or desirable short- and long-term outcomes like energy, efficiency, happiness, maturation, depth of personality, and responsiveness to social and moral predicaments. These tradeoffs challenge the assumption of universalism in biomedicine and raise questions about the consequences of our willingness to use medications, not only to treat crushing depression, but also for the myriad forms of distress that may signal problems with our way of life.

THE SILENCE OF PROZAC IN JAPAN

Hakuin Zenji used to say to his disciples:
"Listen to the sound of the Single Hand."
—Isshu Miura and Ruth Fuller Sasaki, *The Zen Koan*

Antidepressants represent one of the great successes of psychopharmacology in the last fifty years. The introduction of new classes of antidepressants, particularly selective serotonin reuptake inhibitors (SSRIS) in the 1980s—of which Prozac is the most famous—is generally recognized to be a significant advance, not because of any greater efficacy, but because these drugs are much easier for patients to take due to fewer side effects. These new medications are widely prescribed and reap enormous profits for the drug companies. From 1989 to 1998 the antidepressant market in leading regions grew by 16 percent.[4]

Japanese are enthusiastic consumers of pharmaceuticals. In 2001 Japanese bought more that $50 billion U.S. worth of retail medications, and this figure does not include the use of various medicines based on traditional Japanese medicine (*kanpo*).[5] Japan also has one of the highest levels of psychiatric services in Asia with more than seven psychiatrists per 100,000 population.[6] Japanese psychiatry descends from German neuropsychiatry of the turn of the twentieth century and is very "biologically" oriented, so there is no problem with employing medications to treat what are understood as biological disorders.

It comes as some surprise, therefore, that until 2001 antidepressants were not widely prescribed in Japan. Indeed, SSRI medications were not even available in Japan until very recently.[7] The first SSRI in Japan, fluvoxamine (Luvox [Solvay]) was introduced in May 1999, and paroxetine (Paxil [SmithKline Beecham]) was released in November 2000. Although some Japanese psychiatrists have obtained SSRI medications themselves in other countries and made them available to their patients, the initial adoption of newer antidepressant agents was very slow. As David Healy remarked, "The antidepressant market here [in Japan] seems very small—it seems amazing that Prozac isn't even on the market here."[8] As of the autumn of 2001, however, the situation was rapidly changing, and sales of the antidepressant paroxetine (Paxil) had reached more than 1 billion yen (almost $10 million U.S.) per month. This rapid change speaks to the malleability of popular culture and professional practice, but the long lag time for the introduction of new antidepressants and widespread diffidence about their use still demands an explanation.

There are many reasons for the initial reluctance of Japanese psychiatrists and patients to use antidepressants in general and to adopt the newer SSRI medications. There are wide variations across countries in the prevalence of depression, and the actual community prevalence of depression in Japan is not known.[9] It is likely, however, that there are many undetected cases among people who do not seek help or who are seen only in medical clinics where they are not diagnosed with depression but with various physical conditions based on the somatic symptoms that commonly accompany depression.

Until recently, psychiatry in Japan has been focused almost exclusively on the inpatient treatment of major psychoses in private psychiatric hospitals. The emphasis on severe disorders reinforces the stigma associated with psychiatric diagnosis and treatment. As a result, patients with milder neurotic or depressive conditions prefer to be seen as outpatients in general internal medicine or "psychosomatic" clinics. Visits to outpatient psychiatry came under the coverage of national health insurance in the mid-1980s, and since then use of outpatient services has increased. Nevertheless, "depressed individuals in Japan often do not visit their family physicians, and if they do they are often told that they just need to relax more."[10] Instead, they often go to internists who deal with "psychosomatic medicine," and estimates are that about 20 percent of patients seen in that setting have depression. There they are likely to receive a diagnosis of a stress-related condition or constitutional sensitivity and be given antianxiety medications, primarily benzodiazepines.

Again, until very recently, Japanese psychiatrists have preferred antianxiety drugs to antidepressants.[11] This reflects the salience of anxiety in Japanese psychology and psychiatry.[12] There is also a tendency to prescribe small doses of antipsychotic medications to patients who have borderline or schizotypal personality traits. This fits with a view, inherited from German psychiatry, of many problems as being related to specific temperaments or character types that are constitutional and that can sometimes be modified by pharmacological interventions.[13]

There are also regulatory and economic reasons for the lack of use of SSRI antidepressants in Japan. It takes a very long time for new medications to be approved by the Ministry of Health and Welfare.[14] This follows on past episodes in which new drugs were withdrawn when it was discovered they had terrible side effects. At present, government regulations require independent demonstrations that the medication is safe and effective in the Japanese population. Thus, drugs must undergo a new randomized clinical trials (RCTs) in Japan. However, it is difficult to conduct RCTs in Japan. Patients and their families have been reluctant to take part. Western medicines are perceived as "strong," harsh, or unnatural, which is a problem particularly when the condition they are supposed to treat is not viewed as severe or life threatening. This perception has been reinforced in the case of SSRIs because of reports of patients experiencing side effects of nausea and other gastrointestinal symptoms.

The high cost of carrying out drug trials in Japan blocks development especially if the potential market seems small.[15] Initially Prozac was not developed in Japan because of the high cost of redoing the clinical trials and the perceived lack of an adequate market. Eli Lilly considered that the market for Prozac in Japan would be so small that the company could not recoup the costs of the trials and evaluation procedure.[16] More recently, a clinical trial of nefazadone (Serzone [Bristol-Myers Squibb]) was abandoned due to the company's pessimistic view of its potential market.[17]

Of course, there is no guarantee that a clinical trial will demonstrate the drug's effectiveness. A clinical trial of sertraline (Zoloft [Pfizer]) was unable to show a therapeutic benefit.[18] Similarly, buspirone (Buspar) was not approved due to a lack of benefit greater than placebo in two multicenter double-blind trials in Japan. There are also institutional problems in how drug trials are carried out in Japan, so that small beneficial effects may not be detected. Collegial relationships and the small size of many hospitals mean that trials often involve many centers, each contributing only a few patients; this leads to too much intersite variation, which can swamp clinical effects.[19] As well, in some studies mildly anxious patients, for whom less benefit of antidepressants might be expected, were included in the trial along with severely ill patients. Indeed, similar studies in Japan have failed to show effectiveness of diazepam (Valium), although evidence from elsewhere is overwhelming that it is more effective than placebo for anxiety.

The use of antidepressants reflects physicians' judgments about which types of problems are appropriately treated by that specific class of medication. This judgment is both an empirical decision about what works and a consequence of how disorders are grouped together or related in psychiatric nosology.

Although biomedicine is based on scientific evidence about the efficacy of different treatments, in actual practice, clinical decisions involve going beyond the available pool of scientific information. They also involve a process of translating information about groups or populations into a course of action for a given individual. Empirically, drugs do not have single effects both because they usually affect several different receptor sites and because specific neurotransmitters in the brain are involved in many different functional systems, which need not correspond to any single coherent category in our folk psychology or notions of human faculties. The brain has spatial structure and connectivity that involve higher levels of organization than those captured by analysis in terms of neurotransmitter systems or receptor sites.[20] As a result, every medication has many different, sometimes competing or contradictory, effects, and the balance of these may differ in different patients. Clinicians' impression as to what works, therefore, is biased on their experience with a particular group of patients and by the weight they give to the different effects of medication.

In addition to these neurophysiological facts, we need to recognize that systems of psychiatric classification are not simply accounts of natural categories in the world but reflect cultural conventions for

LAURENCE J. KIRMAYER

how to group problems together in ways that make sense.[21] Depression, as "melancholia," has a long tradition in the West as a socially meaningful category of distress—although its social and moral significance has changed radically over the years.[22] Accordingly, depression occupies a central place in psychiatric nosology, and the discovery of effective drug treatments reinforced that category. The gradual recognition that many other conditions are also helped by antidepressants (including panic disorder, generalized anxiety, obsessive-compulsive disorder, body dysmorphic disorder, hypochondriasis, chronic pain, and many other conditions), far from challenging the definition of depression as the prototype for a core category, has led to efforts to widen the definition to cover a broad spectrum of disorders.[23] Of course, the mere fact that a treatment is effective for many conditions does not prove they are all related—aspirin is good for pain due to many different conditions as well as for inflammation and fever from literally thousands of different diseases.

For Japanese psychiatrists, problems with anxiety and social relatedness form more natural prototypes for constructing families of disorders.[24] In the 1920s Shoma Morita described a range of anxiety related problems, including neurasthenia, hypochondriasis, and social phobia, that he felt reflected common underlying problems of excessive self-awareness (*toraware*) and effortful striving to fit in to social situations.[25] Morita developed a specific form of treatment, modeled on the meditative practices and philosophical orientation of Zen Buddhism, aimed at leading patients to "let go" and accept things as they are (*arugamama*).[26] He found the treatment effective for a wide range of conditions.[27] Although Morita therapy has never been more than a marginal practice in Japan available at a few centers, its underlying assumptions and perspective are more influential, as they fit well with cultural and professional notions of personality as rooted in constitution but as modifiable through disciplined practice.[28]

American psychiatric nosology and practice has had increasing influence on Japanese psychiatric theory and practice in recent years.[29] Some younger Japanese psychiatrists have had training in the United States and are promoting models of practice similar to those standard in North America. Nevertheless, there are many features distinctive to Japanese psychiatric practice.

From a Japanese point of view, the popularity of Prozac as a medication that "changes personality" is related to the importance of competition in American society. Dr. Sakai Kazuo, director of Stress Care Hibiya Clinic, was quoted in the *Tokyo Shimbun* newspaper (August 18,

1999): "[Prozac] is a drug that can transform minus thinking to plus thinking. It became known as a drug that gives confidence to the unconfident, and was used by a TV-caster. This drug swept away negative images associated with psychiatry. In the background of this popularity, there seems to be a need to live 'tough' in the competitive American society."

This enthusiasm for SSRIs is found among some younger psychiatrists, but it has not penetrated the general practice of psychosomatic medicine, where "if it comes to a choice between anxiolytics and antidepressants, the anxiolytics still win out."[30]

In an interview with David Healy, Toshi-Hiro Kobayakawa, a leading Japanese psychopharmacologist, invokes differences in the Japanese genetic constitution and value system to account for the slow adoption of SSRIs:

> Genetically the Japanese seem to have less mental disease than in the west. In the west, people are always preoccupied with themselves, whereas the Japanese system is much more modest and cooperative—people work together much more. Against this background, amphetamines are much more of a problem than are the benzodiazepines; we are much more sensitive to the changes, the exaggerations of behaviour, produced by the amphetamines. The behaviour of people in the west is already more exaggerated, so amphetamine-induced problems are less obvious, but here amphetamine abuse is a big social problem and it interacts with criminal activities. Sedative agents are seen as much less of a problem in Japan. . . . There is something of a preference for an agent that will be sedative rather than arousing, like, perhaps, Prozac.[31]

In his remarks, Kobayakawa slides easily between notions of a distinctive constitution and of a unique value system that characterizes the Japanese. There may well be important genetic differences in drug metabolism and response to psychopharmacological agents, but in most cases these remain to be established.[32] The confident assumption and promotion of the idea that Japanese are fundamentally different from non-Japanese is a form of cultural essentialism common in Japan in a genre of literature termed Nihonjinron that celebrates the uniqueness of the Japanese people.[33] Many Japanese are comfortable with the notion that they are somehow distinct from other peoples, not only because of their culture but in the very substance of their brains and bodies.[34] This popular literature on the distinctiveness of the Japanese is ideologically driven and can be more mystifying than illuminating.

LAURENCE J. KIRMAYER

Nevertheless, the striking differences in the practice of psychiatry in Japan raise interesting questions about the universal applicability of psychiatric nosology and treatment. Are these differences merely a result of the persistence of old-fashioned methods of diagnosis and treatment in Japan, due to a reluctance to introduce new medications? Or is there something deeper going on that challenges some of our assumptions about emotional health and illness?

A substantial literature in cultural psychiatry challenges the universality of the categories of disorder enshrined in official psychiatric nosologies like DSM-IV and ICD-10.[35] While there is some evidence that the cardinal symptoms of depression co-occur as a cluster or syndrome in many disparate cultures, it is equally clear that there are culturally distinctive symptoms related to idioms of distress and ethnophysiological ideas. To the extent that depression is a psychological process involving specific cognitions and interpretations of one's self-efficacy and self-esteem, culturally shaped notions of the person and core values related to success and failure, and attachment and loss, will influence both the clinical syndrome of depression and its course over time.

HOW CULTURE MAKES A DIFFERENCE

The roots of the term "culture" lie in cultivation, in working the natural world to make it yield what is of sustenance and value to human beings.[36] Notions of what is natural and what is cultivated or man-made are central to how cultures define themselves. Of course, the binary opposition of nature and culture allows different value systems. Those who embrace scientific progress herald the potency and purity of the newest drug. Those who long for simpler times put their faith in what is "natural." It is common in North America, for example, to hear people endorse herbal remedies as natural—implying that the natural is good, gentle, and harmonious, while chemically engineered medications or designer drugs are harsh, dangerous, and insulting to our bodies. The metaphors of nature and culture, natural and engineered, stand in for whole systems of values.

Ironically, cultures "naturalize" their most central values and commitments; what seems to be simply natural is, in fact, culturally constituted. This is particularly powerful in the domain of psychology. Ethnopsychologies—cultural models of how people work, of the functioning of thoughts, feelings, and motives for action—are commonly presented as "human nature." This appeal to nature tends to elide the cultural and historical origins of our concepts. Cross-cultural comparison unmasks this naturalizing tendency and allows us to critically examine our assumptions in the construction of human nature. Accordingly, in this section I consider some ways in which the regulation of affect in interpersonal relationships and concepts of self and personhood differ between Japan and the United States.

The Regulation of Affect

Individuals differ in temperament or personality. Placed in similar situations, some people are more cheerful, while others are more dour and pessimistic; some are outgoing and self-confident, while others are shy and retiring. These differences reflect both hereditary factors and early developmental experiences. Many features of depression or milder dysphoria may reflect exaggerations of these temperamental traits. If so, SSRI medications may act to change these traits or propensities and hence, in a sense, modify the individual's personality. This might account for the report by some patients given SSRI medications that they feel better than they ever have, indeed, "better than well."[37] The possibility that medication might alter personality raises interesting ethical issues. But these issues depend crucially on the social context that defines desirable and undesirable personality traits.

Cross-cultural research suggests that the ideal personality traits as well as the threshold of intensity at which traits are viewed as problematic may differ across cultures.[38] As a result, one society's enhancement of personality can be another's provocation. Something like this may occur with Prozac, where the extroversion, gregariousness, and pushiness that typify the life of a salesman in the United States may be associated with inappropriately brash and insensitive social behavior in Japan (frequently lampooned on TV). Instead, Japanese value calmness, containment, and sensitivity to the social hierarchy, which are associated with fitting in and helping social interactions unfold smoothly.

As David Healy has pointed out, the more common response to the "better than well" claim is to invoke not a dimensional view of personality but a categorical view that assumes that people who do not have conventional symptoms of depression but who do respond to SSRIS with greater well-being did, in fact, have undiagnosed variants of depressive disorder (like chronic low-grade depression or dysthymic disorder or pathological shyness and inhibition).[39] This assumes that de-

LAURENCE J. KIRMAYER

pressed mood or social anxiety and inhibition always have the same meaning and implications across cultures for the health and functioning of the person. There is reason to believe that this is not the case.

Culture has effects across the lifespan on the neural systems, psychological representations, and interactional patterns that constitute affect. Cultural ideologies, institutions, and practices provide the context and rules for interactional processes that underlie complex emotions. Cultural variations in the composition of the family, maternal-infant interaction, and child rearing practices all prime and shape affect systems. Emotion "display rules" and body practices regulate socially acceptable and deviant patterns of emotional expression. Culture provides categories and a lexicon for emotional experience, making some feelings salient and others more difficult to articulate. Culture sets limits of tolerance for specific emotions and strong affect; it also provides lay theories and strategies for managing dysphoric mood, anxiety, or depression. Each of these ways in which culture may influence the regulation of emotion has potential implications for the expression of dysphoric affect in clinical settings.

In many cultures, disturbances of mood, including depression and anxiety, are not viewed as mental health problems but as social or moral problems. Painful feelings provide socially and morally important information about intolerable or disvalued circumstances, altering a moral landscape and providing a moral compass. Pathological moods are recognized not simply by their painfulness, negativity, intensity, or duration but by their social inappropriateness and lack of responsiveness to context.

In her ethnographic study of menopause in the late 1980s, anthropologist Margaret Lock found that Japanese women frequently mentioned irritability as a problem, but they rarely mentioned depression.[40] This was in marked contrast to Canada, where depression was a common symptom and, indeed, a reason for doctors to prescribe hormone replacement therapy as well as antidepressants. Part of the difference has to do with the cultural meaning of menopause, but there are also differences related to the understanding of depressed mood in general.

In Japan, depression has wide recognition as a notion, but there is no exact translation of the English word. Japanese terms usually glossed in English as "melancholy" or "depression" include *yuutsu* (related to grief but also to gloominess of spirits and weather); *ki ga fusagu* (one's *ki* or vital energy is blocked or clogged); *ki ga meiru* (*ki* is leaky); *shizumu* (low in spirits); and *inki* (*ki* is yin rather than yang—

that is, *in* rather than *yoo*). These general notions of loss or block-age of energy lead to bodily as well as mental manifestations: "The subjective experience of melancholy or depression in Japan is not associated primarily with the head . . . or simply with affective states but is a much more diffuse concept that manifests itself as numerous physical changes including headaches, chest pain, a 'languid' body, or a 'heavy' head."[41] This notion of energy fits with a Japanese concept of the body not as a machine (which can be functioning efficiently or broken down) but as an organic process in constant exchange with the environment.[42]

Sadness and grief are positively valued experiences—indeed, there is a whole aesthetic surrounding the acknowledgment of imperma-nence and loss.

> Feeling sad and reacting sensitively to losses, particularly of loved ones, is an idea that has a singular appeal in Japan. The theater, a range of literature and indigenous popular songs, traditional and modern, positively wallow in nostalgia, sensations of grief and loss, and a sense of the impermanence of things. People cry freely (by North American and northern European standards) about separa-tion and lost loved ones, but at the same time they seem to draw strength from these experiences, to tighten their bonds with those who remain among the living, and to reaffirm group solidarity. . . . Unlike anger and irritability, which both disrupt harmony and threaten the social order, sadness, grief, and melancholy are ac-cepted as an inevitable part of human life and even welcomed at times for their symbolic value, as a reminder of the ephemeral na-ture of this world. An association between melancholy and the weather reinforces sad feelings as natural and unavoidable and hence as states not induced solely through human exchange.[43]

In recent years the notion of depression as disorder or disease has gained currency in Japan. If the behavior of an individual is seriously impaired, he or she may be labeled as having *utsubyoo* (depressive ill-ness). But milder forms of depression are not generally recognized as an affliction. In an effort to make the diagnosis more acceptable, de-pression is often said to be like a cold, an acute and transient ailment, but one that affects the *kokoro*, the heart-mind. According to Japanese psychiatrist Yutaka Ono, the analogy is helpful, as it suggests the bio-logical, treatable, and everyday nature of depressive illness, but it is misleading in that depression can be more severe and long term and require ongoing treatment.[44] Based on her fieldwork, Margaret Lock insists, "I do not believe . . . that the Japanese assigned much negative value to transient feelings of being 'down.' Even when depression becomes more persistent, the culturally conditioned mode of experiencing and expressing such sensations is by means of a somatic idiom that attaches little or no stigma or moral approbation. Furthermore, the very concepts of 'psyche' and 'repression' have little recognition beyond a rather narrow professional circle of psychiatrists and psychologists."[45] Given the positive value of sadness derived from acknowledging impermanence, loss, and imperfection, any medication that mutes the individual's capacity to experience ordinary sadness and grief would be damaging to his or her moral personhood, aesthetic sensibility, and spiritual development.

Concepts of Self and Personhood

In the 1920s, French sociologist Marcel Mauss pointed out that all societies have implicit notions of what it is to be a person.[46] Personhood is not necessarily conferred in equal measure on all individuals or in quite the same way at different developmental stages (infancy, childhood, adulthood, and old age). Outside legal or juridical settings, the cultural concept of the person is implicit and encoded in moral notions of what makes a person good or bad, in ethnopsychological notions of mental health and illness, and in social norms for gender roles and developmental tasks.

European and American notions of the person have strongly influenced psychiatric theory.[47] The American concept of personhood centers on an ideology of individualism.[48] A person is the locus of private experience, of rational choice and preference, and of unique agency and action. Our notions of health and illness, implicit in psychiatric nosology and in everyday clinical judgments about patients, are based on this notion of the person and corresponding ways of narrating and experiencing the self.

The Euro-American self is described as egoistic, individualistic, or independent and valuing the exercise of idiosyncratic choice and agency, extroversion, and instrumental efficacy. In contrast, Japanese (or more widely, Asian) concepts of personhood emphasize the interconnectedness of self and others, focus on social context, and encourage the person to engage in self-criticism, to improve the self through sympathy for others in relationship.[49] The development of these culturally divergent forms of the self may be mediated by the ways in which everyday mundane situations are collectively defined and negotiated, that is, by the tacit rules and practices of everyday social life. These are encoded as prototypical scenes, situations, and scripts or narratives.

Traditionally, Japanese notions of the person are relational and stress interdependence rather than independence.[50] This has implications both for how health is measured and for hierarchies of values. Japanese cultural practices and lay theories of the person affect basic ways of construing or constructing the self and managing adversity. Specifically, there are differences in processes of critical self-appraisal, attachments or investment in the self, and long-term commitments to relational self-improvement.

Thus, Japanese tend to avoid attributing positive outcomes to themselves and emphasize interdependence.[51] Success tends to be attributed to the group; failure, to one's own limitations. Failure leads to reorienting oneself to the group rather than protecting oneself by attributing failure to the actions of others.[52] American health psychology would deem this a recipe for demoralization and depression. The conventional wisdom has it that to avoid depression, one should attribute success to one's own efforts and failure to external exigencies. But there is no evidence that this contrary strategy has negative effects for the Japanese. Instead, conformity to cultural values supports the person's adaptation and well-being.

Health psychology has other versions of this optimal person that also reveal cultural biases. Consider the construct of "hardiness," a concept introduced by Salvatore Maddi.[53] Hardy individuals are optimistic and resilient; they are active copers, adjust well to adversity or obstacles, and are able to continue to pursue their own goals and to modify them appropriately, without getting unduly anxious or depressed, when aspects of a situation are insurmountable. They exhibit a deep sense of commitment and purpose in life, flexibility in adaptation to changes, and a sense of personal control over events. In short, they are rugged individuals. Throughout Maddi's account of hardiness, American middle-class values of expressive individualism hold sway.[54] The hardy hero takes on the world as something to be mastered, bested, and transformed to his or her individual liking.

It is revealing to compare Maddi's account of psychological health to other notions of personhood and the good life. While Maddi emphasizes the ability of healthy individuals to control the environment to make it conform to their agenda, control in Japan tends to be diffused throughout the work or family group while responsibility is held by each individual vis-à-vis the group.[55] For Maddi, "to do something new is developmentally more valuable than persisting in the old."[56] Few masters of traditional arts in Japan would agree. Doing things more slowly, traditionally, the "hard" way, has its own merits.[57]

Based on research conducted around 1990, Gordon Mathews discusses the importance in everyday Japanese moral discourse of the concept of *ikigai*, a term that can be glossed as "that which makes one's life seem worth living."[58] Japanese men tend to find *ikigai* in work or family, while women locate it in their relationships with family and children. The focus on *ikigai* in public discourse was surely a reflection of the relative wealth of Japanese society and increasing longevity. While surveys indicate that most men find *ikigai* in their work, this may be insufficient, and some articles warned that reporting work as *ikigai* may be associated with depression.[59] Japanese recognize the danger of being a workaholic (*waakahorikku*) and that overextension at work can lead to death (*karoshi*). The economic downturn after the burst of the bubble economy has been associated with an increase in suicide, particularly among middle-aged men facing reversals at work.[60]

Contemporary Japanese concepts of the person have their roots in older traditions but underwent profound transformations in the transition to an urban industrial and bureaucratic society from the late 1800s onward.[61] Classic Anglo-American works on self-development, notably *Self-Help* (1882) by Samuel Smiles, were best sellers in Japan and extremely popular among the samurai in the 1870s. The Meiji reformation attempted to bring Japan into a modern economic exchange with the West by dismantling the feudal structure and allowing people to pursue different vocations. No longer were social status, wealth, and honor decided by birth and divine order. In this context, the translation of *Self-Help*, with its famous first line, "Heaven helps those who help themselves," supported the attack on hereditary status.[62]

The Japanese translator of *Self-Help*, Nakamura Keiu, was a Confucian scholar in the employ of the Tokugawa house. He visited Victorian England and was deeply impressed by its wealth and power, successes he attributed to a national character based on values of hard work, prudence, and self-restraint.[63] In the original Anglo-American versions of this character ethic, "accomplishment and advancement were the products primarily of individual virtues of character, hard work, diligence, frugality, perseverance, attention to detail, and so forth. Developing these virtues was a task for the individual himself, and they and his performance were depicted as the sole factors determining achievement and advancement. . . . The character ethic largely ignored interpersonal relations."[64]

Of course, the text rooted in British individualism was given a Japanese Confucian reading. "For the translator, Nakamura Keiu, the chief attraction of *Self-Help* was this assertion by Smiles: 'National progress is the sum of individual industry, energy, and uprightness, as national decay is of individual idleness, selfishness, and vice.'"[65] Thus, Nakamura kept the country in the foreground of his translation. "Individualism and individuality were two important concepts appearing in *Self-Help* that were not well articulated in either Confucian or samurai traditions."[66]

> Both Confucianism and Buddhism had a concept of the self and gave much attention to the subject but they did so in the context of suppressing or negating the self. Confucianism was used most often to link the individual to social or political entities and to encourage contentment with the status quo. It denied the intrinsic worth of all individuals, an essential element for individualism, and called instead for recognition of differential worth according to age, sex, rank, or relationship. . . . It generally did not recognize a sphere of privacy in which the individual was free to pursue his own way.[67]

In contrast to the emphasis on self-actualization and self-efficacy in American individualism,

> the Japanese archetype of growth looks more to "personality"—I use the word here not in its psychological meaning but in the sense of a capacity for human relationships. Perhaps this could be called a people-centered worldview; it is not "sociocentric" in the sense of being primarily attuned to society as an abstract structure of roles. In the Japanese view, we enter into relations with others not from animal weakness but for human strength. . . . The lifelong struggle is to carry out one's responsibilities to others without diminishing one's playful responsiveness toward them. The Japanese cultural nightmare is to be excluded from others, for this renders one unable to do anything with his "personality."[68]

Japanese personhood is thus located not so much in a private inner theater as in the space between individuals where a web of obligations, respect, and mutual nurturance can be developed. Japanese forms of self-discipline can be understood as responses to the "endless need to reconcile the claims of different circles of human attachment."[69] What happens when we take a drug that alters our sensitivity to these circles of attachment, that changes the valences or values assigned to particular options, and that alters our sensitivity to subtle social cues? While it may be helpful in the United States to assert oneself whatever the wishes or discomfort of others, in Japan to barrel along without attending to others would be a path to social suicide.

BUDDHIST TRANSFORMATIONS OF THE SELF

Hifu datsuraku shitsukushite
Tada ichi shinjitsu nomi ari

[Now that I've shed my skin completely
One true reality alone exists]
—Isshu Miura and Ruth Fuller Sasaki, *The Zen Koan*

In an influential paper, anthropologist Gananath Obeyesekere argued that depression was a culture-bound construct. He claimed that he had friends and colleagues in Sri Lanka who met many of the criteria for a major depressive episode, in terms of bleak and negative thoughts, but who were not disabled.[70] Instead, as practitioners of Buddhism, their "symptoms" of depression were cultivated as indications of the unfolding of wisdom. Obeyesekere's claims are somewhat rhetorical and overstated in that the Buddhist practitioners he described were not suffering from the sort of anguished and derailing depression that brings people to a psychiatrist. Such severe depression is recognized in Sri Lanka and would surely interfere with meditation as well as the performance of social roles demanded of Buddhist monks. But Obeyesekere's argument is worth considering seriously in relation to the milder forms of everyday unhappiness for which SSRIs may sometimes be prescribed.

The human condition is inevitably marked by illness, aging, loss, and death. Buddhism teaches that suffering comes not directly from these realities but from our incessant efforts to deny or ignore them and to hold on to what we desire while shutting out what we dislike. This ignorance and grasping is the real cause of suffering. Liberation begins with acknowledging this reality and meditating on impermanence or emptiness to achieve wisdom and compassion through non-attachment. Buddhism offers many techniques to achieve this transformation of the self, not simply as a philosophical principle, but as an experiential reality. The most basic of these techniques are the various forms of meditation developed in different Buddhist traditions. The aim of meditation is not greater effectiveness in the everyday world — although, tellingly, this is how Buddhism is often packaged, especially in the West. The ultimate goal is enlightenment: transcending ordinary confusion and suffering through understanding that the self is an illusion.

Although the insights of Buddhism are usually hard-won achievements after long meditative practice and study, there is within many traditions a notion of sudden enlightenment or transformation. Zen Buddhism, one of several families of approaches to Buddhist practice developed in Japan, has many stories of practitioners suddenly achieving enlightenment. Often these were associated with situations that revealed the ordinary working of mind even as they completely undermined usual modes of constructing experience. These dramatic moments of transformation were captured in brief stories or sayings called koans and used by others later as objects of meditation or philosophical study to advance their own practice.

Koans form part of several systems of meditative practice. The story, poem, or fragment of dialogue works as a focus of meditation not simply because of its density and opacity but because the koan is interpreted in terms of a larger religious system. While in Rinzai Zen the koan was used to induce an enlightenment experience through intensification of doubt, confusion, blockage, and confutation leading to breakthrough, in medieval Soto Zen koans were studied as "models of truth or idealized statements of truth."[71] Koan study "encapsulated Zen transcendence in tangible forms, expressed it in concrete performances, and allowed it to be communicated easily to monks, nuns, and laypersons."[72]

Koans were used in Rinzai Zen to produce sudden enlightenment (*kensho*).[73] It is instructive, therefore, to compare the process of koan meditation with drug-induced changes of mind. Both drugs and meditation offer the possibility of sudden transformations of experience. But the path through koans involves hard work and mental application. Only when the student's mind is exhausted by paradox and the Zen master's rejection of facile answers does the koan accomplish its work of confuting or short-circuiting rationality. This then leads to a sudden reorganization of consciousness and experience.

The sudden transformations celebrated in Zen seem to promise an end to suffering no less abrupt than what is achieved by medication. If the goal of self-development is simply to feel better, to not overreact to adversity, or to be less attached to one's own pleasure and pain, then a pharmacological path toward enlightenment would seem close at hand. If not, what precisely is the difference between the fruits of meditation and the quick fix of medication? What sort of transformative agent is a drug? Can it have more far-reaching effects than a change in mood?

To begin to answer these questions, we must see both meditation and the taking of medication as what Ludwig Wittgenstein called "forms of life." In a course of spiritual practice, years are devoted to training, with consequences for many aspects of the self and the person's understanding of the world. Zen practice is culturally and historically situated.[74] The religious experience of practitioners and the wisdom they achieve depend on the cultivation of specific cultural knowledge. "The koan genre, far from serving as a means to obviate reason, is a highly sophisticated form of scriptural exegesis: the manipulation of 'solution' of a particular koan traditionally demanded an extensive knowledge of canonical Buddhist doctrine and classical Zen literature."[75] Each meditative experience has meaning within a larger moral system, which it confirms and extends. The insights achieved through practice transform the self and at the same time reaffirm the larger spiritual community with whom the practitioner remains in dialogue. So, even where there is an apparent rupture or radical transformation of identity and experience, the experience fits a narrative template that is familiar and consolidates the individual's understanding.

Similarly, the act of taking a drug has meanings that are embedded in larger cultural systems of value and practice. The difference between drug and meditation, thus, lies not only in their physical effects on the nervous system but also at higher orders of organization involving longer temporal spans, accessing of memories, and alterations of modes of awareness and self-construal—a whole head full of cultural particulars. The resultant larger pattern or structure of experience is expressed through and embodied in narratives of the self.

PHARMACOLOGY AND THE NARRATIVE
CONSTRUCTION OF THE SELF

> Not thinking of good, not thinking of evil, just this moment, what is your
> original face before your mother and father were born?
> —Thomas P. Kasulis, *Zen Action/Zen Person*

Many strands of contemporary philosophy, cognitive science, and literary studies have converged on the notion that the self is a narrative construction. This means that our sense of being a person, of having a point of view, an idiosyncratic history, and a social position and a trajectory along which we move toward an unknown but variously imagined horizon of the future is brought into being and maintained by stories we tell ourselves and others. This powerful idea has reshaped our understanding of memory and identity and, more recently, has begun to shift approaches to moral and ethical reasoning.

Taking an antidepressant alters the narrative self in at least three different ways: (1) it changes the bodily feeling and stance that subserve our metaphorical constructions of self, for example, by making us feel more upright and energized; (2) it provides a new inner agent to which to attribute our feelings and actions and a new actor ("the drug") in the social world, with significance to others; and (3) it may reshape our empathic response to others and so alter the fabric of social life itself.

A drug that alters mood exerts a bias on our self-narrative by changing the topography and dynamics of our emotional response to events. Emotions govern our access to specific memories, the stance or position we take vis-à-vis others, and our sense of what is important. Narratives of self are anchored in a cultural logic of emotion. A shift in mood or a change in emotional reactivity to other persons and events, therefore, can radically reshape the form and content of our narratives of self.

A second way that drugs alter the narrative of self is through the attributions we make for our actions. We may understand our behavior as chemically biased or determined and so claim we could not act otherwise. Alternatively, finding that a drug helps us, we may evaluate other people's predicaments in these terms, wondering why they do not simply take the drug to feel better.

Finally, drugs may change the sensitivity of neural systems that subserve various aspects of social behavior in ways that can alter the nature of social life itself. The enhancement of serotonergic systems, for example, may make an individual more likely to exhibit dominant be-

LAURENCE J. KIRMAYER

havior in social interactions.[76] This, in turn, will be reflected in our self-narratives. For example, if medication makes us feel the pain of others less acutely, we may view them as overreacting to their predicaments and as being fundamentally different from ourselves.

Our ability to feel empathy with others and to respond to their plight depends on our capacity to feel vicarious emotion, understand another's predicament, and respond with emotionally appropriate action. Vicarious emotion (e.g., feeling sad when encountering someone who is sad) depends on the power of another's facial expressions, gestures, speech, and contextual cues to evoke a parallel emotional response. Complex emotions, however, also involve the ability to appreciate the causes and consequences of our feelings, and this aspect of empathy depends on imaginative reconstruction of another's life world and predicament. Emotion and imagination form a feedback loop in which each drives the other to a more complete re-creation of the other's experience. Finally, our ability to distinguish between our own experience and that of another, to achieve a level of detachment, allows us to understand the other's predicament as distinct from our own and hence respond to another in terms of what he or she needs rather than what we ourselves would find comforting.

We need a full range of affective responses to empathize with others and so to understand and respond to their predicaments. Too little emotional responsiveness also may prevent accurate empathy. Too much emotional responsiveness may lead us to overreact to others and lose sight of their feelings in the drama of our own reactions. Persistent moods of depression or euphoria (as seen in bipolar disorder, for example) make it hard to track another person's feelings. Clearly, drugs that alter our mood and emotional responsiveness to others may influence our capacity for empathy. They may render us insensitive to the feelings of others so that we are unable to know what they feel. Alternatively, drugs may make us too sensitive to others' feelings and so unable to think clearly about another (or even to differentiate their pain from our own), and this, too, might impair our moral sense.

The sociomoral consequences of medication (or, for that matter, of psychotherapy) may be difficult to see because we focus on the individual and not on interactions in characterizing depression and good functioning.[77] We tend to view our social world as a given and not malleable or constantly evolving as the outcome of micro-interactions. As well, we are constantly engaged in rationalizing or justifying our actions in terms of socially acceptable ideologies. So any impact that drugs may have on our weighing of social situations is likely to be hidden or discounted by this process of narrative smoothing and rationalization. To see this impact requires that others close to us hold up a mirror—one into which we may not wish to look.

A view of the self as a narrative construction leads naturally to the importance of community (however loosely it is defined). Narratives are, in the first instance, stories told to someone in social context. The others from whom we learn and to whom we tell and retell the stories that define and locate us include our intimate relations, family, and friends but extend through the nested circles of community to wider social institutions and through media to global networks. Part of characterizing a narrative and understanding its meaning involves identifying its multiple sources or influences and its intended and actual audiences. To a large extent, it is the response of the community in which we live that determines whether our story makes sense or nonsense, whether our values lead us to health and happiness or to rejection and ruin. As a result, the form of narratives depends on cultural notions of the person. Even such basic qualities of self-narratives as coherence, continuity, and intelligibility differ according to cultural templates for the self.

This dependence on culture and community means that there is a logical circularity between narratively constructed selves and the moral systems that sustain them. This circularity, in turn, raises the problem of moral relativity: If any story we choose to live becomes our moral compass, we have no way of knowing where we are except within a story, and no way of choosing between stories except from within the one that already defines the moral options. One way to escape the arbitrariness this implies is to make claims for the authenticity or integrity of the self. This usually invokes some form of essentialism in which there is a real or true self that stands above or behind the multiplicity of possible selves invented by the stories we tell others and ourselves. This real self was there at the beginning. Unlike the selfless "original" self invoked in Zen koans such as the epigraph for this section, the "true" self of American folk psychology is closely tied to a version of personal history that provides a counterstory to redress all the ways we feel we have been wronged by others. At the same time, the true self usually closely conforms to one of a few cultural templates for the person and the good life. Far from an original self, this true self is a culturally shaped moral aspiration.

Against the fiction of the true self we can array the many possible selves we would like to be, the person we are supposed to be, the person we "really" are in some higher or larger or ultimate frame. These may all be opposed to the person we are judged to be by others based on our personal history and trajectory. But the traces of our personal acts cannot and should never be erased in the process of re-creation. Owning up to our past is the basis on which moral action is built. Here, then, is one of the most worrisome implications of the chemical reconfiguring of our selves: that it might reinforce our tendency for selective memory of our past deeds and their impact and so undermine the possibility of moral accountability, reparation, and integration.

The danger of forgetting and the healing power and aesthetic value of sadness, grief, and melancholy are strikingly illustrated in the novels of W. G. Sebald.[78] In *The Rings of Saturn*, for example, the narrator tells of his own profound depression and then recounts a meandering walk through the English countryside punctuated by a series of vignettes from the lives of friends, acquaintances, and historical figures with whom he feels a kinship. The episodes are linked by a process of "free association" located not in the individual psyche but in the landscape itself. The reader's uncertainty about what is fact and what is fiction is amplified by the slightly out of focus photographs that accompany the text. All of Sebald's stories wander about an unspoken absence at their center, tracing the contours of a more profound loss, both personal and collective, in the cataclysms of the last century. Sebald's novels are anti-antidepressants that produce their own strange exaltation through calling us to the hard moral work of remembering.

ENVOI: GLOBALIZATION AND THE
MONOCULTURE OF HAPPINESS

Despite the great popularity of SSRI antidepressants in North America and Europe, most of these medications have not yet been introduced in Japan. To a large extent this reflects the general difficulty in obtaining government approval for new drugs. However, there are also specific reasons why the newer antidepressants have been slow to reach the Japanese market. Clinical trials of some SSRI antidepressants in Japan have found limited efficacy or excessive side effects. There may be much depression in the general population that is not recognized or treated as such owing to a different tradition of posology and organization of the health care system. Most patients with dysphoric mood in Japan are seen in specialty medical care, complain of physical symptoms, and are treated with anxiolytic medications. As well, some of the effects of medications like fluoxetine (Prozac) that are viewed as beneficial in the United States, such as increased extroversion and ebullience, may be less valued in everyday life in Japan, since they contravene social norms for calmness and deference in interpersonal interactions. Dysphoria itself may be given positive social meanings as yielding enhanced awareness of the transient nature of the world.

This example from Japan illustrates how the personal and social value of the effects of medication depends on prevailing cultural ideologies of the person. These ideologies are implicit in narratives of the self in illness and health. The effects of a drug are not just on the level of mood but on the narrative fabric of the self. This narrative is evaluated by both laypeople and clinicians in terms of a moral calculus based on social norms and cultural values. However, any characterization of cultural differences in terms of local norms of conduct and ideologies of the person must be set against the forces of globalization in which multinational pharmaceutical corporations are working to redefine normal mood and mental health on a global scale.

The pharmaceutical industry strongly influences physicians' prescribing practices, the direction of research, and even the debate on ethical issues in treatment. Millions of dollars are spent on advertising, gifts, and salespeople who, often on specious grounds, convince physicians to prescribe newer, more costly medications in favor of generic compounds.[79] More insidiously, the pharmaceutical industry has become the major source of funds for clinical trials of new treatments for psychiatric disorders: "As government after government fails to provide their nonprofit independent granting agencies with sufficient resources to meet society's growing demand for high-quality evidence, the drug industry, with its inescapable competition between health and profit, pays and calls the tune for more and more RCTs."[80] As a result, the generation of new evidence on which to base rational medical care is controlled by economic interests: "Knowledge in psychopharmacology doesn't become knowledge unless it has a certain commercial value. The survival of concepts depends on the interests with which they coincide."[81] The selective generation of knowledge frames the field of "evidence-based medicine." The range of alternatives available in clinical decision making is constrained by these larger economic forces. As a result, we are left with an illusion of free choice among a highly limited set of "reasonable" options. Critical analysis of this situation may be compromised by the fact that drug companies also sponsor and support programs in biomedical ethics.[82]

Pharmaceutical corporations and the psychiatric profession are working hand in hand to popularize the notion of depression as a medically treatable disease. There has been an aggressive medicalization of the problem of depression in developed countries like Japan in recent years. This vision has been extended to developing countries through programs like the World Health Organization's Nations for Mental Health, a program largely supported by Eli Lilly and other pharmaceutical companies. In the shantytown of Independencia on the outskirts of Lima, Peru, in 1999, colorful posters described the ten warning signs of depression and urged readers to see their doctor and ask for the latest SSRI by brand name. Professional autonomy thus rides the tail of marketing.

There is a global monoculture of happiness in which we are all enjoined to work to achieve the good life, which is understood to reside in being free of pain, completely comfortable, and ready and able to acquire and consume the greatest quantity and variety of the newest goods and fashions. The rapidity with which the notion of depression and the use of antidepressants are taking hold in Japan may reflect the belated recognition and treatment of a long-standing problem from which many have suffered. It may also reflect a profound transformation of cultural modes of understanding and responding to personal and social problems, with far-reaching effects on the concept of the person and the conduct of everyday life.

Few would argue that crippling depression should be recognized and treated effectively. The concern is about the wider and more prevalent forms of dissatisfaction and distress that may be sensitive indicators that something is wrong not with the individual's psyche but with the social world. The riches of modernity bring their own problems and pathologies rooted in excesses of choice and change, overwork, overstimulation, time pressure, and dislocation.[83] In place of the familiar suffering of privation, people in wealthy nations suffer from misery in the midst of plenty due to a sense of relative deprivation and a loss of connectedness to family and community. Our sense of dysphoria and depression may point to problems not in brain chemistry but in the way we live. The study of cultural difference and diversity provides alternative vantage points from which to consider the moral choices implicit in the mundane practice of taking a pill to feel better.

NOTES

I would like to thank Elizabeth Anthony, Kal Applbaum, Carl Elliott, Junko Kitanaka, Margaret Lock, Furnitaka Noda, Masayuke Noguchi, Yutaka Ono, Osamu Tajima, and Simon Young for helpful comments on earlier versions of this essay. The opinions expressed—as well as any errors and omissions—are my own.

1. Peter D. Kramer, *Listening to Prozac* (New York: Viking, 1993).

2. David Healy, *The Antidepressant Era* (Cambridge, Mass.: Harvard University Press, 1997), 160.

3. M. C. Nussbaum, *The Therapy of Desire: Theory and Practice in Hellenistic Ethics* (Princeton: Princeton University Press, 1994).

4. *IMS Health*, April 4, 2000.

5. M. Lock, "Japanese Psychotherapeutic Systems: On Acceptance and Responsibility," *Culture, Medicine, and Psychiatry* 5 (1981): 303–12.

6. O. Tajima, "Mental Health Care in Japan: Recognition and Treatment of Depression and Anxiety Disorders," *Journal of Clinical Psychiatry* 62, suppl. 13 (2001): 39–44.

7. Some Japanese psychiatrists obtained SSRI antidepressants overseas and made them directly available to their patients.

8. D. Healy, *The Psychopharmacologists III: Interviews by David Healy* (New York: Oxford University Press, 2000), 287.

9. L. J. Kirmayer and D. Groleau, "Affective Disorders in Cultural Context," *Psychiatric Clinics of North America* 24, no. 3 (2001); Tajima, "Mental Health Care in Japan."

10. D. Berger and I. Fukunishi, "Psychiatric Drug Development in Japan," *Science* 273 (1996): 318.

11. Tajima, "Mental Health Care in Japan."

12. L. J. Kirmayer, "The Place of Culture in Psychiatric Nosology: Taijin Kyofusho and DSM-III-R," *Journal of Nervous and Mental Disease* 179, no. 1 (1991): 19–28. A culture-specific form of social phobia, *taijin kyofusho*, continues to be a focus of attention in the Japanese medical literature with more than 200 abstracts on the diagnosis published in 1999, compared with fewer than 100 on depression; see Tajima, "Mental Health Care in Japan."

13. J. Kitanaka, *A History of Psychiatry and Discourse about Social Pathology in Japan: Bibliographic Essay* (Montreal: Department of Anthropology, McGill University, 2000).

14. This cautiousness does not extend to all drugs. The sexual potency enhancing drug sildenafil (Viagra) was introduced in Japan in 1999, within a year of its release in the United States and just six months after Pfizer applied for approval.

15. Berger and Fukunishi, "Psychiatric Drug Development in Japan."

16. Ono Yutaka, personal communication, October 26, 1999.

17. Tajima Osamu, personal communication, October 24, 2001.

18. Among other psychiatric medications, clozapine (Clozaril) was not accepted due to agranulocytosis, although a new clinical trial is in progress

at a limited number of facilities; buproprion (Wellbutrin [Glaxo Wellcome]) received U.S. approval in 1989 but is not in development in Japan; and venlafaxine (Effexor [Wyeth-Ayerst]) had U.S. approval in 1994 and is currently in development in Japan.

19. Berger and Fukunishi, "Psychiatric Drug Development in Japan."

20. Indeed, the tendency to talk about specific chemical systems in the brain (e.g. "serotonergic systems," which use the neurotransmitter serotonin and are preferentially affected by SSRI medications) is a sort of neo-humoral theory that, in its tendency toward sweeping generalization, hearkens back to ancient Greek notions of the bodily humors; the link between black bile and dysphoria is attested to in the origins of the term "melancholia"; see Jennifer Radden, ed., *The Nature of Melancholy: From Aristotle to Kristeva* (New York: Oxford University Press, 2000).

21. L. J. Kirmayer and A. Young, "Culture and Context in the Evolutionary Concept of Mental Disorder," *Journal of Abnormal Psychology* 108, no. 3 (1999): 446–52.

22. S. Jadhav, "The Cultural Construction of Western Depression," in *Anthropological Approaches to Psychological Medicine*, ed. V. Skultans and J. Cox (London: Jessica Kingsley, 2000), 41–65; Radden, *Nature of Melancholy*.

23. In fact, there is evidence that depression and anxiety are closely related (see K. B. Kendler, A. C. Heath, N. G. Martin, and L. J. Eaves, "Symptoms of Anxiety and Symptoms of Depression: Same Genes, Different Environments?," *Archives of General Psychiatry* 44, no. 5 [1987]: 451–57) and that bipolar disorder and schizophrenia may share a common diathesis (see D. Blacker and M. T. Tsuang, "Contested Boundaries of Bipolar Disorder and the Limits of Categorical Diagnosis in Psychiatry," *American Journal of Psychiatry* 149, no. 11 [1992]: 1473–83). Even the broad structure of existing psychiatric nosology, therefore, is still contentious.

24. Kirmayer, "Place of Culture in Psychiatric Nosology."

25. S. Morita, *Morita Therapy and the True Nature of Anxiety-Based Disorders (Shinkeishitsu)* (1928; reprint, Albany: State University of New York, 1998).

26. David K. Reynolds, *Morita Psychotherapy* (Berkeley: University of California Press, 1976).

27. F. I. Ishiyama, "Current Status of Morita Therapy Research: An Overview of Research Methods, Instruments, and Results," *International Bulletin of Morita Therapy* 1 (1988): 58–84.

28. K. Kitanishi and K. Kondo, "The Rise and Fall of Neurasthenia in Japanese Psychiatry," *Transcultural Psychiatric Research Review* 31, no. 2 (1994): 137–52; Y. Ono and D. Berger, "Zen and the Art of Psychotherapy," *Journal of Practical Psychiatry and Behavioral Health* 1 (1995): 203–10.

29. Y. Honda, "DSM III in Japan," in *International Perspectives on DSM III,*

ed. Robert L. Spitzer, Janet B. W. Williams, and Andrew E. Skodol (Washington, D.C.: American Psychiatric Press, 1983), 185–201.

30. Toshi-Hiro Kobayakawa as quoted in Healy, *Psychopharmacologists III*, 286–87.

31. Ibid.

32. K. M. Lin, "Biological Differences in Depression and Anxiety across Races and Ethnic Groups," *Journal of Clinical Psychiatry* 62 (2001): 13–21.

33. Peter N. Dale, *The Myth of Japanese Uniqueness* (New York: St. Martin's Press, 1986).

34. For an extreme example, see Tadanobu Tsunoda, *The Japanese Brain: Uniqueness and Universality* (Tokyo: Taishukan, 1985).

35. J. E. Mezzich, L. J. Kirmayer, A. Kleinman, H. Fabrega, D. L. Parron, B. J. Good, K. M. Lin, and S. M. Manson, "The Place of Culture in DSM-IV" *Journal of Nervous and Mental Disease* 187, no. 8 (1999): 457–64.

36. Terry Eagleton, *The Idea of Culture* (Malden, Mass.: Blackwell, 2000).

37. Healy, *Antidepressant Era*, 53; Kramer, *Listening to Prozac*.

38. J. Paris, "Social Factors in the Personality Disorders," *Transcultural Psychiatry* 34, no. 4 (1997): 421–52.

39. Healy, *Antidepressant Era*.

40. Margaret M. Lock, *Encounters with Aging: Mythologies of Menopause in Japan and North America* (Berkeley: University of California Press, 1993).

41. Ibid., 222.

42. Lock, "Japanese Psychotherapeutic Systems"; E. Ohnuki-Tierney, *Illness and Culture in Contemporary Japan* (Cambridge: Cambridge University Press, 1985).

43. Lock, *Encounters with Aging*, 222–23.

44. Personal communication, October 26, 1999.

45. Lock, *Encounters with Aging*, 223.

46. Marcel Mauss, *Sociology and Psychology: Essays* (London: Routledge and K. Paul, 1979).

47. A. D. Gaines, "From DSM-I to III-R: Voices of Self, Mastery, and the Other: A Cultural Constructivist Reading of U.S. Psychiatric Classification," *Social Science and Medicine* 35, no. 1 (1992): 3–24.

48. Robert Neelly Bellah, *Habits of the Heart: Individualism and Commitment in American Life* (Berkeley: University of California Press, 1985).

49. Takie Sugiyama Lebra, *Japanese Patterns of Behavior* (Honolulu: University of Hawai'i Press, 1976); Nancy Ross Rosenberger, *Japanese Sense of Self* (Cambridge: Cambridge University Press, 1992).

50. G. DeVos, "Dimensions of the Self in Japanese Culture," in *Culture and Self: Asian and Western Perspectives*, ed. A. J. Marsella, G. DeVos, and F. L. K. Hsu (New York: Tavistock, 1985), 141–84; Takeo Doi, *The Anatomy of Self: The*

Individual Versus Society (Tokyo: Kodansha International, 1986); S. Kitayama and H. R. Markus, "The Pursuit of Happiness and the Realization of Sympathy: Cultural Patterns of Self, Social Relations, and Well-Being," in *Culture and Subjective Well-Being*, ed. E. Diener and E. M. Suh (Cambridge, Mass.: MIT Press, 2000), 113–61; Lebra, *Japanese Patterns of Behavior*; Rosenberger, *Japanese Sense of Self*.

51. J. R. Weisz, F. M. Rothbaum, and T. C. Blackburn, "Standing Out and Standing In: The Psychology of Control in America and Japan," *American Psychologist* 39, no. 9 (1984): 955–69; F. Rothbaum, J. Weisz, M. Pott, K. Miyake, and G. Morelli, "Attachment and Culture: Security in the United States and Japan," *American Psychologist* 55, no. 10 (2000): 1093–1104.

52. Situations of overt competition, however, evoke self-enhancement in studies of Japanese students.

53. S. R. Maddi, "On the Problem of Accepting Facticity and Pursuing Possibility," in *Hermeneutics and Psychological Theory*, ed. S. B. Messer, L. A. Sass, and R. L. Woolfolk (New Brunswick: Rutgers University Press, 1988), 182–209.

54. Bellah, *Habits of the Heart*.

55. H. Azuma, "Secondary Control as a Heterogeneous Category," *American Psychologist* 39, no. 9 (1984): 970–71; Weisz, Rothbaum, and Blackburn, "Standing Out and Standing In."

56. Maddi, "On the Problem of Accepting Facticity and Pursuing Possibility," 184.

57. D. Kondo, "Multiple Selves: The Aesthetics and Politics of Artisanal Identities," in Rosenberger, *Japanese Sense of Self*, 40–66.

58. Gordon Mathews, *What Makes Life Worth Living? How Japanese and Americans Make Sense of Their Worlds* (Berkeley: University of California Press, 1996), 5.

59. Ibid., 16.

60. Tajima, "Mental Health Care in Japan."

61. E. H. Kinmouth, *The Self-Made Man in Meiji Japanese Thought: From Samurai to Salary Man* (Berkeley: University of California Press, 1981).

62. Ibid., 10.

63. Ibid., 21.

64. Ibid., 12–13.

65. Ibid., 20.

66. Ibid., 27.

67. Ibid., 332.

68. David W. Plath, *Long Engagements: Maturity in Modern Japan* (Stanford: Stanford University Press, 1980), 217.

69. Ibid., 219.

70. G. Obeyesekere, "Depression, Buddhism, and the Work of Culture in Sri Lanka," in *Culture and Depression*, ed. A. M. Kleinman and B. Good (Berkeley: University of California Press, 1985), 134–52.

71. William M. Bodiford, *Soto Zen in Medieval Japan* (Honolulu: University of Hawai'i Press, 1993), 213.

72. Ibid., 143.

73. Isshu Miura and Ruth Fuller Sasaki, *The Zen Koan: Its History and Use in Rinzai Zen* (Kyoto: First Zen Institute of America in Japan, 1965), 95.

74. R. H. Sharf, in "The Zen of Japanese Nationalism," in *Curators of the Buddha: The Study of Buddhism under Colonialism*, ed. D. S. Lopez Jr. (Chicago: University of Chicago Press, 1995), 139, argues that the popularity of Zen in the West had much to do with the similar problem of relativism that emerged from the encounter with the diversity of religious practices:

> Philosophers and scholars of religion were attracted to Zen for the same reason that they were attracted to the mysticism of Otto, James and Underhill: it offered a solution to the seemingly intractable problem of relativism engendered in the confrontation with cultural difference. The discovery of cultural diversity coupled with the repudiation of imperialist and racist strategies for managing cultural difference, threatened to result in the "principle of arbitrariness," the notion that there is no necessary reason for us to conceive of the world one way rather than another. In mysticism intellectuals found a refuge form the distressing verities of historical contingency and cultural pluralism; by invoking a *sui generis* nondiscursive, unmediated experience they could gracefully elide problems of ontological reference.

75. Ibid., 108.

76. D. S. Moskowitz, G. Pinard, D. C. Zuroff, L. Annable, and S. N. Young, "The Effect of Tryptophan on Social Interaction in Everyday Life: A Placebo-Controlled Study," *Neuropsychopharmacology* 25, no. 2 (2001): 277–89.

77. Thomas E. Joiner and James C. Coyne, *The Interactional Nature of Depression: Advances in Interpersonal Approaches* (Washington, D.C.: American Psychological Association, 1999).

78. Winfried Georg Sebald, *Austerlitz* (New York: Random House, 2001); Winfried Georg Sebald and Michael Hulse, *The Emigrants* (New York: New Directions, 1996); Winfried Georg Sebald and Michael Hulse, *The Rings of Saturn* (New York: New Directions, 1998).

79. A. Wazana, "Physicians and the Pharmaceutical Industry—Is a Gift Ever Just a Gift?," *Journal of the American Medical Association* 283, no. 3 (2000): 373–80.

80. D. L. Sackett and J. H. Hoey, "Why Randomized Controlled Trials Fail

LAURENCE J. KIRMAYER

but Needn't: A New Series Is Launched," *Canadian Medical Association Journal* 162, no. 9 (2000): 1301–2.

81. Healy, *Antidepressant Era*, 176.

82. C. Elliott, "Pharma Buys a Conscience," *American Prospect* 12, no. 17 (2001): 16–20.

83. Zygmunt Bauman, *Globalization: The Human Consequences* (Cambridge: Polity Press, 1998); B. Schwartz, "Self-Determination: The Tyranny of Freedom," *American Psychologist* 55, no. 1 (2000): 79–88.

FINANCIAL DISCLOSURE

Lawrence Kirmayer has received lecture honoraria from GlaxoSmith-Kline.

Prozac for the Sick Soul

In Mark Salzman's novel *Lying Awake*, a nun faces an unusual and troubling dilemma. Sister John of the Cross, a contemporary Carmelite, has for a number of years received intense and profound religious visions. Prior to these visions, her life as a nun was not marked by any special connection with God but instead seemed to have been what her namesake, the sixteenth-century Christian mystic St. John of the Cross, described as a "dark night of the soul." With the end of this spiritual desolation, Sister John feels her life is finally spiritually fulfilling: "Nothing was changed, yet everything was changed. Compared to this, she felt as if she had been sleepwalking all her life. 'God is here,' she answered."[1] Yet her visions are also accompanied by severe migraine headaches, and she is bidden by her superiors to seek medical assistance. Sister John's physician discovers a small meningioma above her right ear that has been triggering temporal-lobe seizures; he explains that these seizures can cause the sufferer to experience the world in a profoundly altered state. This diagnosis enjoins Sister John to regard her visions, the central source of meaning in her life, as the symptoms of a biological disease. The salient drama of Salzman's novel surrounds Sister John's decision of whether to submit to the simple operation that would remove the meningioma and thus relieve her of the seizures.

Salzman's novel draws upon a familiar motif in the modern worldview: the difference between religiosity and psychopathology. A few weeks ago, a medical student on her psychiatry rotation spoke to me about a woman who was being involuntarily kept in the hospital. The woman's primary symptom was that she was praying unceasingly. The health care professionals who committed her were concerned that she would not be able to care for herself on the bitter winter streets of Chicago. The student was troubled by the idea that she was responsible for trying to cure the woman of her religiosity. What if the various medications that the woman was taking resulted in a complete cessation of her praying? I confess to being perturbed by these kind of cases. I know that in another interpretive community, such behavior would be the mark of religious genius. In their study of the difference between "spiritual experiences" and "psychopathology," Mike Jackson and K. W. M. Fulford concluded the distinction is not so much biological as it is hermeneutic, for events interpreted as "psychotic" by medical professionals were viewed by the individuals and by those in their community as being "spiritual in nature and benign in their effects."[2] Sister John's visions only become a medical concern when she is treated for her headaches. Without the accompanying headaches (or the order by her superiors to get medical attention), Sister John would quite possibly have continued to see herself and to be seen by others as a religious prodigy and not as a medical patient.

DEPRESSION AS SPIRITUAL CALL

The conflict between religion and medicine has received a new wrinkle in recent years due to the advent of a generation of psychiatric medications called selective serotonin reuptake inhibitors (SSRIs). Known by such brand names as Prozac, Paxil, Zoloft, and Celexa, these drugs have had a profound impact on the treatment of a number of mental illnesses, especially obsessive-compulsive disorders and depression. Yet aspects of these drugs have disturbed a number of critics.

Perhaps the most well-publicized objections have come from Peter Kramer, a psychiatrist whose 1993 book *Listening to Prozac* was a national best seller. While describing fascinating case histories from his own practice, Kramer thoughtfully explores the impact that SSRIs may have on one's sense of self. For example, he documents his care of "Tess," whose personality radically changed after taking Prozac; she became more confident and more socially at ease. According to Kramer, Tess remarked that, reflecting on her previous life, it felt as if she had been depressed her entire life. This observation causes Kramer to wonder who the "real" Tess is, an issue that becomes even more confusing when, after stopping Prozac, Tess asks Kramer to prescribe it again because without it, " 'I am not myself.' "[3] Kramer also describes his treatment of "Hillary," a woman who suffered from anhedonia, the inability to experience pleasure. According to Kramer, "She had no passion, no enthusiasm, no drive, no initiative, just a sort of lazy passivity grounded in her indifference to the pleasures of life."[4] As Kramer came to know her, he found that Hillary did not exhibit any significant "depressive symptoms," and he concluded that her main problem was "an inability to understand what the fuss was all about."[5] After a series of trials on Prozac, Hillary finally sustained a cure from her anhedonia. Suddenly she found life filled with things to enjoy; she began dating and going to the theater and to concerts and movies. Kramer emphasizes that Hillary was not manic on Prozac and that her behavior and enthusiasm for life seemed "appropriate."

Cases like Tess's and Hillary's make one wonder, From what has the patient been cured? Philosopher Carl Elliott expresses concern that SSRIs may be alleviating patients of existential alienation;[6] he finds the stories of Tess and Hillary troubling because Kramer's patients' angst may be an appropriate response to the late twentieth-century human condition. For Elliott, one of the pitfalls of viewing existential alienation as a psychiatric malady is that the framing of the problem results in a predictable solution. Psychiatry gauges the success of its interactions through the degree of psychic well-being produced in the patient. If alienation occasions a decrease in psychic well-being or social performance, then it is viewed as "something to be eliminated. It is a psychiatric complaint."[7] Elliott considers this emphasis on well-being as the ultimate goal to be of questionable merit; he argues that because psychiatry views all human experiences in terms of psychic well-being, it cannot consider alienation as a potential good in human life.

Compare Hillary's case to that of a young man who was brought to a psychiatrist by his father. From the perspective of an outsider, the young man appears to be leading a very successful life. He is financially secure, has a happy marriage, and is physically healthy. Yet recently he has become obsessed with death, sickness, and old age, and like Hillary, he does not find life pleasurable. Even the recent birth of his first child did not seem to bring him joy. The psychiatrist prescribes Prozac for the man. Two months later, on a follow-up visit, the man reports that he has been relieved of his obsessive thoughts and is finding life pleasurable again. As the years go by, the man becomes an extremely successful leader in a large corporation and an important figure in his local community, especially his church. Although I have taken a few liberties, I have essentially "modernized" the religious myth of the Buddha. Legend has it that when the Buddha was born, his father was informed that he would grow up either to be a great political leader or a great religious figure. Trying to ensure that his son became the former, the father shielded the prince from the tragedies of life. The son, however, could not avoid being overpowered by the tragic truths of life: that we must all suffer from old age, disease, and death. He abandoned his wealth and his family in search of

TOD CHAMBERS

spiritual enlightenment. Would the Buddha on Prozac have remained with his family to lead a less enlightened life?

ZEN AND THE ART OF ANXIETY

American Buddhists themselves have been asking this very question. In an article on Prozac in the American Buddhist journal *Tricycle*, Judith Hooper wonders if the Buddha was "in the grip of deep depression" when he made the decision to leave his family. "Is it possible to see in Shakyamuni's behavior hints of the warning signs in medical pamphlets—'Have you lost interest in life? Experienced changes in appetite or sleep patterns? Stopped socializing with friends?' Was Buddha the sixth century B.C.E. equivalent of the depressed housewife who refuses to get dressed, comb her hair, or cook a meal?"[8] In her conclusion, however, Hooper suggests that one of the problems with the scenario of a "cured" Shakyamuni is that it assumes that he was depressed according to our contemporary understanding of that concept. Possibly, she suggests, "there was then—and always will be—a distinction between a spiritual crisis and a psychological crisis."[9]

In *The Science of Happiness: Unlocking the Mysteries of Mood* (2001), Stephen Braun tells the story of Lou Anne Jaeger, for whom Prozac became a religious trial. Jaeger had suffered from mental illness throughout her life. In college, she was prescribed antidepressants (the pre-SSRI generation) that alleviated her depressions, though episodes reoccurred periodically and included thoughts about suicide. She was eventually put on Prozac, and as with Kramer's patients, her life turned around. She separated from her husband, advanced in her career, and began practicing Buddhism. During her early practice of *zazen* (Zen Buddhist meditation), she felt that she could make do without medication and tried weaning herself from the drug. But during an intense four-day meditation retreat, she began to suffer extreme anxiety and depression and afterward commenced taking Prozac again. Jaeger eventually concludes that she was wrong to believe that meditation could allow her to control her moods. She originally had thought that increasing her Buddhist practice would decrease the need for an antidepressant and, therefore, that the medication was "artificially" keeping her from deepening her religious practice.

Another American Zen Buddhist, Jennifer Green Woodhull, also initially struggled over the issue of taking SSRIs. In her reflections, Woodhull makes the same distinction as Hooper between spiritual and psychological problems. She begins her narrative by juxtaposing what she characterizes as a time when "meditation and medication went to war in my mind": "I am a committed Buddhist of ten years' standing. Every day I swallow 125 mg. of Zoloft. It wasn't an easy decision. And it has changed my life."[10] After moving to Alaska from Colorado, Woodhull, for the first time in her life, was not able to secure work or establish friendships. She responded to this difficult situation by turning to Buddhist teachings, "only to find it eclipsed by my despair."[11] When she started experiencing severe shortness of breath, she consulted a psychiatrist, who recommended she take an antidepressant. Woodhull was shocked by this suggestion. She thought that taking medication for an acute episode may be appropriate, but as an ongoing part of her life, it was a potential danger to her spiritual practice, which required "an uncontaminated mind." Instead Woodhull increased her religious practice. For two years Woodhull suffered from depression, refusing medication but not finding relief through her religious beliefs or practices. When she returned to Colorado, she rethought her position against taking antidepressants and accepted a prescription for Zoloft. She describes her life as having changed in both "subtle and profound" ways now that she is a practicing Buddhist on an SSRI. She contends that she still "suffers," for as Buddhism teaches, this is the nature of existence, but she declares that "the pain of existence no longer absorbs my attention."[12] Because Woodhull separates "the brain" from "the spiritual entity that is mind," she views "medicating a malfunctioning mind" as equivalent to receiving any other medical treatment for the body. In other words, the problem is once again essentially categorical: though psychological crisis and spiritual crisis may look the same, they are two different beasts. Is the crisis you are undergoing a catalyst for spiritual rebirth or simply an obstacle to spiritual growth? The distinction between physical or psychological pain and existential or spiritual pain provides an important rationale for accepting some degree of SSRI use. Yet it remains difficult to discern how the semiotics of the two differ in appearance. How is the expression of existential pain different from the expression of psychological pain?

In *The Three Pillars of Zen*, Buddhist teacher Philip Kapleau includes a series of contemporary accounts of "enlightenment." In most of these first-person accounts, the narrators recall the reasons they initially became interested in practicing Buddhism. An early April entry in the diary extracts of a forty-six-year-old American ex-businessman reads, "Belly aching all week. Doc says ulcers are getting worse. . . .

Allergies kicking up too. . . . Can't sleep without drugs. . . . So miserable wish I had the guts to end it all." [13] Later the same month, after listening to some lectures on Buddhism, he writes, "Zen philosophy isn't ridding me of my pain or restlessness or that damn 'nothing' feeling." [14] Five years of intense Zen practice eventually lead the narrator to an experience of enlightenment; his last entry reads, "Feel free as a fish swimming in an ocean of cool, clear water after being stuck in a tank of glue . . . and so grateful." [15] A thirty-five-year-old Canadian housewife recalls that although she had an "ideal childhood," she began to have "recurrent periods of despair and loneliness which used to seep up from no apparent source, overflowing into streams of tears and engulfing me to the exclusion of everything else." [16] After years of practicing Buddhism, she finally attains a profound moment of enlightenment. "The days and weeks that followed were the most deeply happy and serene of my life. There was no such thing as a 'problem.' Things were either done or not done, but in any case there was neither worry nor consternation. . . . For the first time in my life I was able to move like the air, in any direction, free from the self which had always been such a tormenting bond to me." [17] Writing in the late 1960s, William Johnston contends that a condition known as "Zen madness" was well known among Japanese doctors. [18] This condition was the result of an "artificial psychosis" created by the intended irrationality of Zen koans, questions that one can only understand upon the attainment of enlightenment. [19] We might surmise that if these individuals were to come to the attention of American psychiatrists today, they would be prescribed an SSRI, not a Zen meditation cushion.

Christians, whose worldview advances a very different relationship to suffering, have also been challenged by the impact of Prozac on their spiritual lives. In their article "The Gospel According to Prozac," Andrés Tapia, Clark Barshinger, and Lojan LaRowe ask, "Can it be that a pill can do what the Holy Spirit or human will could not?" [20] The authors illustrate this problem with cases similar to those presented by Kramer. Elisa Walters awakened each day with the same thought: "I want to die." A devout Christian, she turned to prayer and spiritual counseling, but none of these traditional responses to her suffering helped. After going on Prozac, she "felt like living again. And I began to experience God like I never had before." [21] Don Timons worked as an executive in an evangelical organization. He vented his long-term fight with depression through bouts of his uncontrolled anger toward his colleagues, continually repenting to God for these episodes and petitioning for help. His depression and anger were not alleviated until he began a course of Prozac; he states that the change is "akin to how I felt during my conversion experience."[22] For the authors, Prozac's effect on these Christians' lives raises central questions concerning how Christians regard the relationship of personality to sin and redemption. They are troubled as well by Kramer's account of a patient who was both clinically depressed and addicted to pornography. Once on Prozac, the patient finds that not only has his depression disappeared, but so has his desire for pornography. Does Prozac take away sin as it takes away depression? This problem illustrates Susan Squier's important observation in this volume that concerns about the use of enhancement technology always return to questions of control, agency, and identity.

PROZAC AND THE RELIGIOUS TEMPERAMENT

In her memoir *Prozac Diary*, Lauren Slater provides a fascinating glimpse into how SSRIs can affect one's religiosity. Slater had suffered from obsessive-compulsive disorder and depression throughout her life, and she was one of the first to try this new generation of psychiatric medications. Soon after she was relieved of her symptoms, she recounts, she went to her bookshelf to select something to read. Most of her books fell in "the disciplines of psychology, philosophy, and theology" and included Søren Kierkegaard's *Fear and Trembling* and Victor Frankl's *Man's Search for Meaning*. "But now, well, now I stood by my bookshelves a little lost. They were full of death and anxiety, the spines seeming to exude cold clouds. I had no desire to read Kierkegaard."[23] Books that at one time had given Slater "clues about ways to live my life" now seemed antiquated to her new sense of self. She became concerned that the drug that had relieved her of her "disabling obsessive symptoms" had also "tweaked the deeper proclivities of my personality. Who was I? Where was I? Everything seemed less relevant—my sacred menus, my gustatory habits, the narrative that had had so much meaning for me. Diminished."[24] This testimony seems to confirm Elliott's worst nightmare: the creation of a happy King Siddhārtha instead of the Buddha. In the December entry of her diary, however, Slater writes, "I am becoming a little bit spiritual, which I'm sure is not a side effect Eli Lilly reports in its literature on Prozac. After work today, I stopped by the bookstore and picked up Merton, a calm Catholic."[25] A February 10 entry consists of two sentences: "A world I might learn to live in. A world I might learn to love."[26] On the fifteenth of that month, Slater discusses her new interest in "contemplation." She has some questions for the late Trappist monk Thomas Merton: "What does it mean, for instance, that my burgeoning contemplative bent does not come directly from God but from Prozac? Might this mean that Prozac is equal to God? This is an awful, awful thought. So turn it around. Primitive cultures often use drugs as a means of accessing their gods. That's better. Maybe Prozac is to the modern world what peyote is to the Indians."[27]

This change in Slater's spiritual orientation reminds me of William James's classification of two types of religious temperament: the way of "healthy-mindedness" and that of the "sick soul." In his Gifford lectures, James argues that there is an intimate relationship between religion and happiness; the happiness that comes from the adoption of religious beliefs is viewed by the believer as demonstration of the truth of these beliefs. James states that the religion of healthy-mindedness is the result of a personality in which "happiness is congenital and irreclaimable,"[28] "a temperament organically weighted on the side of cheer and fatally forbidden to linger . . . over the darker aspects of the universe."[29] The cosmological perspective of the healthy-minded is that the world is, in essence, good, and only our ignorance makes it appear otherwise. James further distinguishes voluntary and involuntary healthy-mindedness. Involuntary healthy-mindedness is a characteristic of persons born to this mindset and thus constitutionally forged to view the world as having essential goodness at its core. Voluntary healthy-mindedness, by contrast, is the result of a philosophical effort to systematically find goodness. Examples of such voluntary systems of healthy-mindedness can be found in the work of Baruch Spinoza, Teilhard de Chardin, and Gottfried Wilhelm von Leibniz.

A populist at heart, James was interested in a contemporary popular movement of voluntary healthy-mindedness called the Mind-cure. This movement emphasized that one is already, in a sense, "saved" but prevented from realizing this fact only by a vestige of our evolutionary past, namely fear. In purging oneself of "fearthought" or the "misery-habit," one will break through to seeing one's essential unity with God. Healthy-mindedness views the human being as fallen not due to some essential, inherent evil but, rather, because of an individual's incorrect worldview.

The way of the sick soul is that of one who is "congenitally fated to suffer from" the presence of evil.[30] From the perspective of these "morbid-minded types," evil and unhappiness do not simply result from our naïveté, but constitute the fabric of the world. This temperament views the healthy-minded as superficially optimistic and unwilling to acknowledge that all our achievements are tainted by sickness and death. This insight results in "religious melancholy," a general disease with all of life; James relates religious melancholy to anhedonia. He understands the sick soul's response to the world as an expression of "the native temperament of the subject," whose character seems innately to posses "a certain discordancy or heterogeneity."[31] For the discordant personality to overcome its melancholy, there must be a radical transformation through a process of unification. Examples of sick souls include Søren Kierkegaard, Leo Tolstoy, and Simone Weil. James's unfamiliarity with Buddhism would have precluded him from using the story of the young Shakyamuni's reaction to sickness, old age, and death as a paragon of this type of melancholy.[32] But the Buddha also exemplifies the manner in which some individuals of this temperament can attain happiness through a dramatic and painful process of unification. James remarks that to those of the sick soul, "healthy-mindedness pure and simple seems unspeakable blind and shallow"; to the healthy-minded, the sick soul's path is "unmanly and diseased."[33]

We should probably maintain a good deal of skepticism toward James's simple division of religious types into only two clear, distinct categories. (I suspect, however, that James, a philosopher fascinated with diversity and pluralism, would have welcomed any expansion of his categories.) These categories may, however, provide a rudimentary vocabulary for understanding the alterations in religious orientation brought about by SSRIs. Prior to taking Prozac, it seems that Slater had the religious temperament of the sick soul. She ultimately achieves happiness not through a dramatic spiritual rebirth but, instead, through the SSRI's alteration of her temperament. Reoriented toward the way of healthy-mindedness, she turns away from the melancholy world of Kierkegaard and toward the calm, contemplative world of Merton.

THE VIRTUE OF RELIGIOUS DIVERSITY

Should we be disturbed by this new orientation? I suspect that James might have found it troubling, for although he wished to remain objective in his description of religious types, he clearly favored the path of the sick soul. In the Gifford series, James devoted only two lectures to healthy-mindedness but spent five on the sick soul. This favoritism may be attributed to James's own personal struggles or to the fact that he was an American thinker. The distinctively American character of James's philosophy can be seen in his implicit valorization of melancholy. Elliott states that "spiritual emptiness, the search for a sense of self, alienation in the midst of abundance" are American traits.[34] Are we a nation that loves the sick soul and thus treasures the intellectual, aesthetic, or religious offspring of the spiritual struggle? Walker Percy—Elliott's own muse on existential alienation—encapsulates this disdain for the orientation of healthy-mindedness when he states, "Consider the only adults who are never depressed: chuckleheads, California surfers, and fundamentalist Christians who believe they have had a personal encounter with Jesus and are saved once and for all."[35] Kramer considers Elliott's promotion of alienation as "a cultural preference for the melancholic over the sanguine."[36]

Comparing Kierkegaard to New Age spiritualists clearly stacks the deck against healthy-mindedness; it is akin to comparing the paintings of Edward Hopper to the paint-by-numbers creations of a retired banker. The West has tended to give greater esteem to those geniuses that struggle for their insights and thus have—in an emblematically capitalist manner—"earned" them. To create brilliant and complex artwork without depression, alcoholism, or at the very least, obsessive nail biting, is akin to having inherited one's wealth. Similarly, religious genius has also been viewed as springing from painful struggle; images of religious conversion portray sudden, powerful turns in individuals' lives, such as Paul being struck down on his way to Damascus, Augustine being bidden to take up the Bible, and Black Elk's transformative vision of the future. But conversion can also occur through a measured intellectual acceptance of a new worldview. The healthy-minded have their own admirable heroes. It seems a far more fit comparison to place Baruch Spinoza alongside Søren Kierkegaard and Aldous Huxley alongside Walker Percy. Healthy-mindedness need not be dull or intellectually suspect.

In his last book, *A Passion for Truth*, Abraham Heschel offers a fairer competition through his portrayal of two important Jewish figures in Hasidism. The book is essentially a personal account of Heschel's own attraction to the healthy-mindedness of Israel Ba'al Shem Tov and the sick soul of Menaham Mendle of Kotzk, the former representing cherished love and the latter, truth.

The Ba'al Shem Tov saw all of life as an opportunity for joy; the sense that some have of God's absence from their lives occurs because "with the palm of one hand upon our eyes, we obstruct our own view."[37] According to this view, if we would only remove this obstruction, we would be always in God's presence. By contrast, the Kotzker rebbe valued "alienation": all of existence seemed "alien" to him.[38] Like Kierkegaard, whom Heschel considers this rebbe's Christian spiritual counterpart, the Kotzker suffered throughout his life from melancholy. Heschel contends that this melancholy may be "a condition that enables a man to see through the falsehood of society and to come upon the burial place where Truth is entombed."[39] These two religious thinkers' mental anguish is not simply the product of personal idiosyncrasy but, rather, represents a latent universal condition of living truthfully in the modern world. If, as James insinuates, one's reaction to evil helps to differentiate the healthy-minded from the sick soul, then the Ba'al Shem Tov and the Kotzker clearly represent differing religious temperaments. The Ba'al Shem Tov taught that evil was merely a "temporary manifestation" of good that lies hidden from our view.[40] The Kotzker saw evil as "a fierce enemy, stubborn and mighty" and insisted that we "must fight it boldly, head on."[41]

In the end, Heschel finds himself unable to choose between these teachers and feels his life richer for having both. "The Ba'al Shem suspends sadness, the Kotzker enhances it," he explains. The sadness brought about by the Kotzker was due to the vigilance one must keep against "the constant peril of forfeiting authenticity."[42] For Heschel, a world that lacked either a passion for truth or a passion for love was seriously impaired. While I am suspect of those who view the healthy-minded to be inferior to sick souls, I do not think a world made up only of Ba'al Shem Tovs is any more desirable than one that only contained Kotzker rebbes. I am not troubled by the way Prozac alters the self toward healthy-mindedness, for I do not think the healthy-minded live any less an authentic religious life than does the sick soul. But I remain concerned that this pharmacological transformation may limit the spiritual and psychological diversity. The value that we should be concerned with is not authenticity but, rather, diversity.

NOTES

1. Mark Salzman, *Lying Awake* (New York: Knopf, 2000), 116.

2. K. W. M. Fulford and Mike Jackson, "Spiritual Experience and Psychopathology," in *Healthcare Ethics and Human Values: An Introductory Text with Readings and Case Studies*, ed. K. W. M. Fulford, Donna Dickenson, and Thomas Murray (Malden, Mass.: Blackwell, 2002), 146.

3. Peter D. Kramer, *Listening to Prozac* (New York: Viking, 1993), 18.

4. Ibid., 224.

5. Ibid., 225.

6. Carl Elliott, "The Tyranny of Happiness: Ethics and Cosmetic Psychopharmacology," in *Enhancing Human Traits: Ethical and Social Implications*, ed. Erik Parens (Washington, D.C.: Georgetown University Press, 1998).

7. Carl Elliott, "Pursued by Happiness and Beaten Senseless: Prozac and the American Dream," *Hastings Center Report* 30, no. 2 (2000): 11.

8. Judith Hooper, "Prozac and the Enlightened Mind," *Tricycle*, Summer 1999, 110.

9. Ibid.

10. Debra Elfenbein, ed., *Living with Prozac and Other Selective Serotonin Reuptake Inhibitors (SSRIs): Personal Accounts of Life on Antidepressants* (San Francisco: HarperSan Francisco, 1995), 202.

11. Ibid.

12. Ibid., 204.

13. Philip Kapleau, *The Three Pillars of Zen* (Garden City, N.Y.: Anchor-Doubleday, 1980), 209.

14. Ibid., 219.

15. Ibid., 239.

16. Ibid., 266.

17. Ibid., 278-79.

18. William Johnston, *The Still Point: Reflections on Zen and Christian Mysticism* (New York: Fordham University Press, 1970), 10.

19. For another perspective on the relation of depression to Buddhism, see Gananath Obeyesekere, "Depression, Buddhism, and the Work of Culture in Sri Lanka," in *Culture and Depression*, ed. Arthur Kleinman and Byron Good (Berkeley: University of California Press, 1985), 134-52.

20. Andrés Tapia, Clark Barshinger, and Lojan LaRowe, "The Gospel According to Prozac," *Christianity Today* (1995), 35.

21. Ibid.

22. Ibid.

23. Lauren Slater, *Prozac Diary* (New York: Penguin, 1999), 28.

24. Ibid., 29.

25. Ibid., 85.

26. Ibid., 93.

27. Ibid.

28. William James, "The Varieties of Religious Experience," in *Writings, 1902-1910*, ed. Bruce Kuklick (New York: Library of America, 1987), 78.

29. Ibid., 81.

30. Ibid., 126.

31. Ibid., 156.

32. Ibid., 466.

33. Ibid., 169.

34. Elliott, "Pursued by Happiness and Beaten Senseless," 8.

35. Walker Percy, *Lost in the Cosmos* (New York: Washington Square Press, 1983), 79, quoted in Carl Elliott, "Prozac and the Existential Novel: Two Therapies," in *The Last Physician: Walker Percy and the Moral Life of Medicine*, ed. Carl Elliott and John Lantos (Durham, N.C.: Duke University Press, 1999), 65.

36. Peter D. Kramer, "The Valorization of Sadness: Alienation and the Melancholic Temperament," *Hastings Center Report* 30, no. 2 (2000): 15.

37. Abraham Joshua Heschel, *A Passion for Truth* (New York: Farrar, Straus and Giroux, 1973), 18–19.

38. Ibid., 202–3.

39. Ibid., 207.

40. Ibid., 40.

41. Ibid., 30.

42. Ibid., xv.

FINANCIAL DISCLOSURE

Tod Chambers owns stock in Eli Lilly, Pfizer, and Teva Pharmaceuticals.

CONTRIBUTORS

Tod Chambers is associate professor of bioethics and medical humanities at Northwestern University's Feinberg School of Medicine. He is the author of *The Fiction of Bioethics*.

David DeGrazia is associate professor of philosophy at George Washington University in Washington, D.C. He is the author of *Taking Animals Seriously: Mental Life and Moral Status* and of numerous articles in philosophy and ethics journals.

James C. Edwards is professor of philosophy at Furman University. He is the author of *Ethics without Philosophy: Wittgenstein and the Moral Life*, *The Authority of Language*, and *The Plain Sense of Things*.

Carl Elliott is associate professor of pediatrics and philosophy at the University of Minnesota Center for Bioethics. He is the editor of *Slow Cures and Bad Philosophers*, coeditor with John Lantos of *The Last Physician*, and the author of *A Philosophical Disease*, *The Rules of Insanity*, and *Better Than Well: American Medicine Meets the American Dream*.

David Healy is reader in psychological medicine and director of the North Wales Department of Psychological Medicine at the University of Wales College of Medicine. He is the author and editor of many books, including *The Antidepressant Era* and *The Creation of Psychopharmacology*.

Laurence J. Kirmayer is director of the Division of Transcultural Psychiatry at McGill University. He is the author of many articles in psychiatric journals and editor in chief of the journal *Transcultural Psychiatry*.

Peter D. Kramer is clinical professor of biomedical psychiatry and human behavior at Brown University. He is the author of *Listening to Prozac*, *Should You Leave*, and the novel *Spectacular Happiness*.

Erik Parens is associate for philosophical studies at the Hastings Center. He has published extensively on the ethical and social questions raised by biotechnological advances. He is also the editor of *Enhancing Human Traits: Ethical and Social Ramifications* and coeditor of *Prenatal Genetic Testing and the Disability Rights Critique.*

Lauren Slater is a clinical psychologist and director of AfterCare Services, a mental health and substance-abuse clinic in Boston. She is the author of *Welcome to My Country, Prozac Diary, Lying: A Metaphorical Memoir, Love Works Like This,* and *Opening Skinner's Box.*

Susan Squier is Brill Professor of Women's Studies and English at the Pennsylvania State University. She is the author of *Babies in Bottles* and *Virginia Woolf and London* and is coeditor of *Playing Dolly, Arms and the Woman,* and *Women Writers and the City.*

Laurie Zoloth is director of bioethics at the Center for Genetic Medicine and professor of bioethics and medical humanities at Northwestern University. She is the author of *Health Care and the Ethics of Encounter* and coeditor of *Margin of Error, Notes from a Narrow Ridge,* and *The Human Embryonic Stem Cell Debate.*

INDEX

STUDIES IN SOCIAL MEDICINE